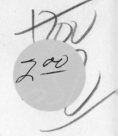
MAKING PEACE WITH FOOD

MAKING PEACE
WITH FOOD

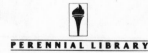

Freeing Yourself

from the Diet/Weight Obsession

REVISED EDITION

SUSAN KANO
DRAWINGS BY LINDA BOURKE

PERENNIAL LIBRARY

Harper & Row, Publishers, New York
Grand Rapids, Philadelphia, St. Louis, San Francisco
London, Singapore, Sydney, Tokyo, Toronto

FIRST EDITION

Designer: Cassandra J. Pappas

LIBRARY OF CONGRESS CATALOGUE CARD NUMBER: 88-45561
ISBN: 0-06-096328-X

93 TI/RRD 10 9 8 7 6

To the joy of
feeling
at home in our bodies and
living
in harmony with our hungers

CONTENTS

ACKNOWLEDGMENTS

When I decided to self-publish this book in 1985, many people feared that I would regret it, myself included. I knew nothing about publishing, the financial risk was substantial, and, statistically, I had an excellent chance of ending up with a garage full of unsalable books. But I tried it anyway, and throughout the long and arduous process, my friends and family offered nothing but encouragement, helping hands, and faith in my ability to beat the odds. I would like to thank them all for their loving support.

I especially thank Emelia Benjamin, M.D., Jennifer Kano, Rev. Cathy Munsey, Eric Tarini, Edith Berman, Judith Coolidge, Denise O'Connor, Linda Doctor, Robin Boots, and Andrea Berman, all of whom helped in the preparation of the self-published edition.

I thank my friend and first editor, Rebecca Shuster, for her careful and insightful editing, and her absolute appreciation of me and my work.

I thank Edward Goodstein, M.S., R.D., who provided extensive comments and suggestions from a nutritionist's perspective.

Above all, I thank my parents, Cyrus and Dorothy Kano. Without their love and generosity I would not have had the emotional or financial resources to self-publish. I am especially grateful to my mother, who not only proofread much of my work, but also honed my writing skills.

Because of the tremendous support I received, my own hard work, and the subsequent enthusiasm of health professionals, readers, and bookstore managers, the self-published version of *Making Peace with Food* became a great success. Only one dream remained to be fulfilled: that of selling it to a "real" publisher. I would like to thank my father-in-law, Joseph Bower, for providing the initial link with Harper & Row; my agent, Deborah Schneider, for turning the link into a contract; and my Harper & Row editor, Janet Goldstein, for offering useful suggestions and respecting my work and opinions.

Most of all, I would like to thank my husband and best friend, Jonathan Bower, for his endless love and support. He encouraged me at every stage, from writing to publishing, selling, and the recent updating and revising. He explained all the financial mysteries I needed to understand (including why the faster sales grow, the more money one has to borrow). And, most important of all, he helped me feel good about myself.

PREFACE

When I completed the original manuscript for *Making Peace with Food* in 1985, I harbored many unanswered questions and fears about the resulting book. I knew that my manuscript was extremely helpful to college-age women because I had tested it with workshop members at the Simmons College Health Center for over a year. But this was a very small and homogeneous sample. What about everyone else? Would it "speak to" people of all ages and sizes? Would the medical/professional community be skeptical of a self-help book written by a former dieter and recovered borderline anorexic?

Over the past three years, an abundance of favorable response has answered my questions and stilled my fears. I have lectured for nutritionists, women's groups, parents' groups, college students, eating disorder groups, and school advisers, and these audiences have provided considerable feedback. I have run workshops that include women of all ages, and members have shared their experiences. And I have received wonderful, thoughtful letters of gratitude and celebration from women of every size and shape, from emaciated to obese. I have also heard from women of many ages, from teenagers to grandmothers. I have heard from yo-yo dieters, anorexics, and bulimics. In short, women from many walks of life, suffering from a wide variety of problems, have felt that I was speaking to *them*, probably because we have all shared so much of the same pain surrounding our bodies, our eating, and ourselves.

On the other hand, I've also heard from those violently opposed to the idea that people can actually be at peace with their eating and their bodies or, horror of all horrors, eat spontaneously! This point of view has been voiced by a number of audience "call-ins" to radio and TV talk shows where I have been interviewed. These people fear that my philosophy encourages poor eating, poor health, self-indulgence, and an additional fifty pounds for all.

My answer is as follows: I encourage my readers to "indulge" in treating themselves well. Of this I am 100 percent guilty as charged. I encourage them to reclaim a natural way of eating that respects their body's hunger signals, to accept and, yes, even *love* their natural size and shape, to celebrate the joy of movement in dance, exercise, or sport, to value *who* they are (not just what they look like), and to feel as good as they can feel and enjoy life as completely as they can.

I find that when people truly reach for these goals, they gradually learn to live well, which includes nourishing themselves well. They take good care of themselves, not out of duty or feelings of guilt, but out of a natural desire to be healthy and happy.

Those who read my book are generally in search of *peace*. They have been suffering with an internal war. Now they want to be at peace with food, with their bodies, and with themselves. They want freedom from the tiresome and painful conflict. *Making Peace with Food* offers a road to that freedom.

"But how free can you really be?" I've repeatedly been asked.

Even as I wrote this book, I often had to force myself to be free. I would remind myself not to feel guilty about eating; I avoided scales like the plague because seeing "the number" triggered negative feelings and thoughts, and I still exercised somewhat obsessively to ward off body anxiety. On the other hand, I never dieted, I always ate whatever I wanted, I rarely overate, I didn't watch or worry about my weight, and my weight was stable. Having been utterly obsessed about my eating and weight not long before, I felt *incredibly* free. And I wasn't sure I could get a lot freer.

Now I realize that I was unduly pessimistic, for today I feel *much* freer. I never need to remind myself not to feel guilty about eating because it never occurs to me to feel guilty. I can weigh myself if I want to, and "the number" has no effect on me. And I no longer exercise obsessively.

How free can you really be?

In my opinion, there are *no limits.* I feel wonderfully free today, but I expect to feel even freer five years from now. I will never be free of the memories of starving, bingeing, watching my weight zoom up, forcing my weight to go down, feeling desperate for food, freezing day in and day out, etc. But time keeps passing and, with it, the shadow and the burden of those memories. Food and eating are no longer problems for me at all, but I keep learning to feel better about my body and myself, which brings even greater freedom and peace.

The letters I have received from readers have truly warmed my heart. There is nothing better than getting a letter from someone you've never met saying, "I feel wonderful! Thank you!" Let me share part of an inspiring letter I received from a college student last November:

> Since I was 12 or 13, I have had a continuous struggle with food and my body. When I read your book last February, I was going out of my mind with food/dieting/body-image problems. From the time I read this book, my whole life has changed. It's incredible. I never diet. I rarely overeat. I exercise regularly because it makes me feel good—not to lose weight. In fact, I was able to successfully exercise on a regular schedule for the first time this summer after reading your book. I feel a million times better about my body and about myself.

Preface

Of course, not everyone has benefited from *Making Peace with Food* in such a dramatic fashion. Nor is it really the book that brings about the transformation, but rather the reader's hard work. I hope that you will find in *Making Peace with Food* a self-affirming, encouraging, and practical self-help program. More important still, I hope that your efforts will bring a sense of greater peace, freedom, and pride in yourself.

I wish you all the best life has to offer.

S.K.
SEPTEMBER 1988

1
THE PROBLEM: POUNDS OF FAT OR PILES OF PAIN?

Do you often think about how "fat" you look? Have you ever thought, "I was bad today—I'll starve myself tomorrow"? Do you repeatedly size yourself up in mirrors (and occasional store windows) despite the fact that your size and shape always look about the same as they did at last inspection? Do you often want to eat something but deny yourself? Have you ever felt full yet desperate to eat?

Years ago, I had to answer "yes" to all of these questions. Many of my friends had to answer the same way. We assumed these aggravations were "inevitable"—that we couldn't afford to stop. But none of us liked it.

If you are struggling to become or remain thin, this book is for you. If you have developed a painful preoccupation with diet, body weight, and shape, I am speaking to you. My goal: to help you *free yourself from the diet/weight obsession.*

Don't get the wrong idea: this is not a "diet book." You have probably tried many diet and exercise programs, only to find that your problems with diet and weight remained. I am not going to send you through that treadmill again. Almost all of the people who buy diet books and go to weight-loss clinics do *not* overcome their problems with diet and weight. In fact, the five-year follow-up records of virtually every diet program indicate that a third to a half of dieters gain back *more* weight than they lose.[1] It is commonly estimated that only 2 to 10 percent lose weight permanently,[2] and even many of these dieters continue to suffer from severe conflicts surrounding their diet and weight. Very powerful and unavoidable causes, many of which are physiological, underlie this problem (see Chapter 2).

Diet books try to answer the insistent questions of a society obsessed with thinness—"How can we lose weight?" "How can we eat less?" "How can we maintain lower weights?"—instead of addressing the question many of us have finally begun to ask: "How can we stop being preoccupied and upset by our eating, body weight, and shape?"

I learned how to control my diet, lose weight, and maintain a very low weight. But after achieving these goals, the real problem remained: unhappiness, dissatisfaction, and pain caused by an obsession with diet, weight, and shape. In fact, my "success" intensified the problem.

My personal experience and pain has been the primary source of motivation and insight for this book. I suffered through three years of dieting, bingeing, and yo-yoing weight (in a 30-pound range) as I struggled to become "model thin." When I thought I had succeeded, I found myself maintaining a weight of under 100 pounds (I'm 5'3"). By then I had stopped getting periods; I felt cold all the time; I suffered from the most severe depressions of my life; and all of my sexual feelings and responses had disappeared. Nonetheless, I clung to this condition through a semistarvation diet and obsessive exercise for almost two years because I was so proud to be thin and in complete control of my diet and weight.

Most of these struggles occurred while I was a college student. My conflicts with diet and weight led me to write many papers on related topics, do my own research, run workshops for women who had eating disorders, and, finally, write my thesis on the development of eating disorders. When I completed this work, I was still keeping my weight below 100 pounds. I knew that I had to stop dealing with the subject of eating

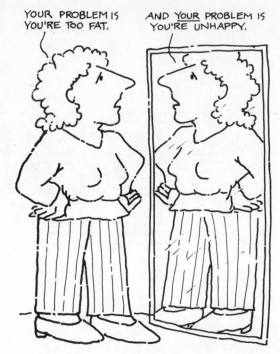

disorders as a researcher and support-counselor, and begin dealing with it as a borderline anorexic who was determined *not* to become a full-fledged anorexic.

During the next two years, I slowly but surely worked through my eating disorder. I gradually let go of strict dietary controls and regained my healthy weight. I remained conscious of my eating and weight, but I ceased to be bothered by them. I ate whatever I wanted to eat and never "dieted," yet my weight was stable. Just three years before, I would have sworn that I could never eat spontaneously without endlessly gaining weight. It was a joy and a relief to let go of my eating disorder and discover that I was wrong.

Most of you have probably heard of eating disorders such as anorexia nervosa and bulimia. You may be wondering whether or not *you* have an eating disorder. Consider these questions:

1. Do you want to become (or remain) slender and lean, or "slimmer" than you are now?

2. Do you feel that *without* dietary controls, which require much self-denial and effort, you would become very fat?

3. Are you tense or anxious about controlling your eating and weight?

4. Is your *self-esteem* affected by the extent to which you maintain control over your diet and weight?

If you answered "yes" to all of these questions, then you have what I would call an

SOME OF THE SYMPTOMS	ANOREXIA NERVOSA	BULIMIA	CHRONIC DIETING
1. Desire to be thin or "thinner"	yes	yes	yes
2. Preoccupation with dietary control; chronic attempts to eat less	yes	yes	yes
3. Preoccupation with eating (chronic hunger, cravings, etc.)	yes	yes	yes
4. Preoccupation with thinness/fatness and distorted body image	yes	yes	yes
5. Low and unstable self-esteem, which is affected by the degree of diet/weight control achieved	yes	yes	yes
6. Fear of losing control	yes	yes	yes
7. Fear of gaining weight	yes	yes	yes
8. Depression, despair, loneliness	usually	usually	often
9. Excessive/obsessive exercising	often	often	often
10. Frequent binge eating	no	yes	sometimes
11. Purging through vomiting, laxatives, or diuretics	sometimes	yes	no
12. 25% or more weight loss	yes	no	no
13. Amenorrhea (no menstrual periods)	yes	often	sometimes

The Problem: Pounds of Fat or Piles of Pain?

eating disorder. Many clinicians would disagree because they only recognize established eating disorders that have more *visible* symptoms. However, I define eating disorders from the "inside out" rather than from the "outside in." Anorexia nervosa and bulimia share a group of core symptoms that cannot be physically observed. These basic symptoms are the shared attitudes, beliefs, and fears of people who have eating disorders. You may not have anorexia or bulimia, yet *think and feel* like people who do. In that case, you probably suffer from what I call "chronic dieting," the most widespread eating disorder of all.

Drawing lines between people who have eating disorders and people who don't is not the most important issue. *If you are at all uncomfortable with the way you deal with your eating and weight, then you have a problem that deserves attention and relief.* You do not deserve to suffer. You need not accept that suffering.

Isn't it interesting, and doesn't it cut close to home, that without the "t," the word "diet" becomes "die"? This is fitting for a number of reasons. First, because uncountable numbers of people have literally died from their efforts to diet down to slenderness: people have died from liquid protein diets; people have died from self-starvation still thinking, even on their deathbeds, that they needed to lose more weight; one of my friends nearly died from a potassium deficiency because of a weight-loss diet. Thus, many people have died and others are dying now because of absurd diets.

Second, dieters all over the Western world are suffering "little deaths" because of their efforts to lose weight. Little deaths are those moments or hours or days when we are focused on an internal struggle between our hunger and our desire to eat and weigh less. We die little deaths every time we are unable to enjoy ourselves because we have eaten too little—when we feel irritable and tired because we haven't had enough to eat. We die little deaths every time we feel annoyed, immobile, and guilty because we've stuffed ourselves half to death. These are little deaths because while we are consumed with that kind of torment, we destroy our ability to love anyone fully, to appreciate ourselves, or to enjoy living.

Worse yet, those of us who are chronic dieters sometimes experience a prolonged "living death." We stop feeling affected by people, situations, and activities. We feel that our lives can no longer touch us inside: everything is flat, nothing is fun, sexual feelings and responses are lost. . . . When experience ceases to touch us, life becomes meaningless. We even begin to ask: "Why bother living?"

I have written this book to help you reclaim the joy of eating in an unconflicted way. You can choose not to diet, and in doing so, choose not to "die yet": not to die a premature death, not to experience the little deaths of a diet/weight preoccupation, and not to experience a prolonged living death.

Many more women than men suffer from diet/weight conflicts and eating disorders; however, these are not exclusively "female problems"—far from it. When I ran workshops at a coed college, men asked for help even though all advertisements were addressed to women. These brave men were part of a much larger group of male sufferers, most of whom were too embarrassed to seek help.

Many chapters of this book can help men who are preoccupied with diet and weight, although it is primarily a book for women.[3] Men and women share many experiences and feelings; however, we are treated differently on the basis of gender. We are brought up differently, we are pressured in different ways, and the messages we receive about our appetites and our bodies are especially different. Within these differences lie the reasons why so many more women than men suffer from diet/weight preoccupation and eating disorders. This is a book for women in that it often focuses on women's experiences—why we, as women, have developed diet/weight preoccupation, and how we, as women, can reclaim our freedom from it.

We are living in the midst of an *epidemic* of diet/weight preoccupations that range from mild concern and anxiety to life-threatening eating disorders. Literally millions of people are struggling with the addictive cycle of bingeing and purging.[4] Chronic dieting is so common that many people think of it as a "normal" condition. Thus, whether you are only mildly troubled by your diet and weight or you are making yourself throw up four times a day, *you are not alone.* You are surrounded, in fact, by people who share your pain.

Some of the causes of this epidemic are physiological, some are psychological, and some are cultural. The cultural causes are a particular challenge because we are constantly bombarded with influences that support the development and maintenance of diet/weight preoccupation and eating disorders.

Nearly everyone in our culture takes part in, and compounds, these harmful influences. Without knowing it, people from all walks of life are supporting the epidemic through things they say and do. In the course of this book, you will learn how to undermine diet/weight preoccupation instead of encouraging it. I have included this training not only because you can help stem the epidemic, but because you must stop supporting it in order to overcome *your own* diet/weight preoccupation.

Sometimes I still fear that I will not be able to let go of the last remnants of diet/weight preoccupation unless I move to a culture that does not encourage it. If the attitudes around us move in the right direction, however, complete freedom will become much easier to achieve. Thus, as *you* work toward freedom from diet/weight preoccupation, you will help not only yourself, but me and millions of other people who share your pain.

I STUDIED THE MANUAL, WHY CAN'T I STEER THE BOAT?

I still remember the first day of my first philosophy class in college. The professor announced that we would be required to hand in file cards filled with personal comments on what we'd read and how it might apply to our own lives and philosophies. One of my classmates confronted the professor with indignation: "The assignment," he complained, "was junior-highish"—an insult to his intelligence. Other students nodded in agreement.

The professor remarked that a semester rarely went by without the same complaint, and then asked, "Do you learn more from direct experience or reading about the same topic?"

"Direct experience," we naturally replied.

"Do you learn more from something you participate in personally or something you observe?"

We agreed that participation was usually better.

"And what do you retain and think about more: things you apply to your personal lives, or impersonal abstractions—like most of what you'll be tested on at this or any other university?"

Once again, the answer was obvious.

"I'm glad you see it that way," the professor concluded. "Now you can also see why I want you to write personally significant comments instead of impersonal analyses, or worse still, notes. If I test your comprehension and retention today, you'll probably forget by tomorrow. I'd rather you left this course with a personal change in philosophy, or at least a personalized view of certain philosophies. Any more questions so far?"

Like my old professor, I encourage you to interact with, think about, and apply information by asking yourself personal questions. I have therefore provided questions (and space for answers) at the end of each chapter. I have no intention of talking down to you through these questions. You have the intelligence and ability to free yourself. This book provides a framework for that process. Think about and answer these questions as you go along. They aren't designed to test your comprehension or memory. They're designed to help you think about what I've said, and to figure out how it applies to you.

I envision you reading and thinking, then writing; reading and thinking, then writing; as you read my book. I strongly encourage you to *write down* your reactions because it will help you comprehend and apply what you read. Written responses will also allow you to go back later and look at your own reactions with a new perspective. Of course, not everyone loves to work through problems on paper. If writing is difficult for you (even when done for no one but yourself), then try discussing what you read and feel with someone you trust—perhaps someone else who would like to read this book. Ideally, do both: write and discuss.

Why is it so important to think, write, and discuss as you read? Because you must take an active role in order to improve your life. You will never free yourself from diet/weight preoccupation simply by reading about it. That would be like trying to learn to sail by reading about sailing every night before bed.

I use this analogy because I once met a man who did just that. He spent uncountable evenings reading books about sailing. Books about sailing around the world in a small boat. Books about sailboat racing. Books about cruising with the whole family. Books about sailing skills and terms. Then he bought a large boat and continued his evening reading. It didn't work. A year later this man still couldn't sail his boat. I imagine him throwing down his books and crying: "I studied the manual! Why can't I steer the boat?"

If you read this book, think carefully, write down your thoughts, and actively work toward your goals, you will be rewarded accordingly. Be aware, however, that it's easy to understand the causes of diet/weight preoccupation, yet continue to suffer from it. Understanding the problem is only the beginning of our struggle: what we "know" tends to be a few steps *ahead* of what we feel and how we act.

Work through this book at your own rate; but *beware of going too fast.* Most of us have been taught to read too fast and process too little. We have been trained to read and absorb and repeat, rather than to question and apply information to ourselves. Questioning and examining personal implications takes much longer than reading. It's a good idea to read a chapter, let it sit for a while (perhaps the rest of the day), review and answer the personal questions on another day, and then process the information through thought

and discussion for a while longer before going on to the next chapter.

This book is designed to help anyone who suffers from conflicts with diet, body weight, and shape, including chronic dieters, bulimics, and recovering anorexics. However, no single program can meet everyone's needs. The workbook pages can help you personalize and apply this program, but you may need further help. If your diet/weight conflicts are severe (or become severe), you should not use this self-help program alone —get professional help as well. If you are very underweight, or making yourself throw up, or abusing laxatives or diuretics, or extremely depressed or upset, you need professional support. In that case, use Chapter 10 to find help as soon as possible. Do not select a therapist at random.

Regardless of whether or not you receive formal therapy, the personal work required to gain freedom from your conflicts with diet

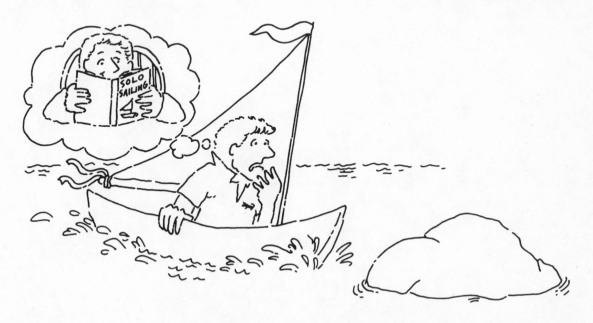

The Problem: Pounds of Fat or Piles of Pain?

and weight will probably be painful. At times you may feel even worse than you felt before you began to work through the problem. Don't give up or be surprised if this happens. Personal growth and progress rarely occur without growing pains, but it's well worth the struggle.

Above all, don't isolate yourself. Be with people, share yourself and your feelings. Let people in. At times it is hard to see, but people are dying to be let in. You are literally surrounded by lonely people. You could break through some of that loneliness, and thereby break out of your own isolation. Wouldn't that be beautiful? All you have to do is reach out.

The information in this book, combined with the things you will think, write, say, and do, will lead you toward freedom from diet/weight conflict. We can dramatically improve the quality of our lives. So—on to happier eating and living!

2

CEASING TO DIET AND DISCOVERING OUR SETPOINTS

You want to be thin but have found that it's not easy to become and remain thin. Since you want to control your weight, you try to control your diet. Thus your preoccupation has two focuses: how much you eat and how much you weigh. We have been taught certain ideas about how and why people gain and lose weight. These assumptions seem logical, but they are inaccurate.

During the last few years, more and more people have questioned basic assumptions about the relationship between diet and weight. The newest evidence supports the theory that each person has a "setpoint weight" that his or her body "prefers" and attempts to maintain, and that this physiologically ideal weight can be well outside the bounds of standard "recommended weights." In *The Dieter's Dilemma: Eating Less and Weighing More*, Dr. William Bennett and Joel Gurin explain that dieting is actually an ineffective means of weight control, an idea that challenges many strongly held beliefs.[1]

Nearly everyone in our culture has tried to lose weight by dieting at one time or another. I assume that you sometimes (or always) restrict your diet because you want to be thin. In order to attain freedom from diet/weight conflict, you must change that pattern. To make this choice, you need to understand why weight-loss dieting* is not only ineffective, but harmful. Let's begin by exposing some of the faulty assumptions that lead us into trouble.

---

* Weight-loss dieting refers to temporary eating programs designed to make one lose weight. They consist of eating less than needed to sustain weight, usually by specifying both the type and the *quantity* of food.

SIX FAULTY ASSUMPTIONS

Faulty Assumption #1:
Fat People Eat More than Thin People

We assume that the more we eat the heavier we'll be, and the less we eat the thinner we'll be. When we see a fat person, we think that she eats too much; when we see a thin person, we think that she must eat a smaller, "more appropriate" amount. In short, we assume that fat people eat more than thin people. This is our first faulty assumption.

A large body of evidence indicates that, in general, fat people do not eat more than thin people. Twelve out of thirteen studies reviewed in *The Energy Balance and Obesity in Man* found the intake of heavier people less than or equal to that of thin people. The remaining study found no difference with one measure and found that the obese ate slightly more with another measure.[2]

Why are so few people aware of the evidence that fat people eat no more (and possibly a little less) than thin people? The answer lies in the researchers' and the public's biases. Many of our attitudes and our industries rely on the assumption that fat people eat more. We don't want to be told, and if told we probably won't believe (or will conveniently forget), that fat people eat no more than thin people.

Many researchers have reported that the eating style of obese people differs from that of thin people. In general, fat people tend to eat faster and respond to circumstances (such as time of day and the availability of food) more than thin people do.[3] On the basis of these studies, researchers concluded that obese people become and remain obese because of a problematic eating style, and in response, behavior modification programs were developed to teach obese people to eat "like thin people."

A few years later, however, it became clear that training dieters to eat like thin people was not producing long-term weight reduction. The primary reason: faulty assumptions. Theorists assumed that abnormal eating styles existed first and caused weight problems. Later studies revealed that fat people tend to have different eating styles because long-term dieting and constant concern about diet and weight changes the way people eat.[4] The so-called "obese eating style" usually develops *after* individuals become chronically concerned with diet and weight. The eating styles do not *cause* the "weight problem." Nonetheless, behavior modification programs based on teaching fat people to eat like thin people still exist and even thrive. The public is so desperate for any promise of weight loss that weight-reduction professionals need not respond to failure. Failure is the norm in their industry.

Since the studies on food intake cited above, many skeptical researchers have sought to contradict the evidence that fat people eat no more than thin people. They have duplicated studies, and they have used many different forms of measurement and observation in a variety of settings.[5] These attempts simply add to the already impressive body of evidence which indicates that fat people, on the average, do not eat more than thin people. Those who maintain that fat people become and remain fat because they eat more have no evidence to support their claim.

Faulty Assumption #2:
A "Slow Metabolism"
Is Just an Excuse

We have been taught that a "slow metabolism" rarely causes a weight problem. We are told to stop using this as an excuse and face the embarrassing fact that metabolism has little to do with it. This is our second faulty assumption.

Normal metabolic differences among people play a crucial role in weight gain, loss, and maintenance. Basal metabolism—the minimum amount of energy needed to carry on vital body processes[6]—varies tremendously. Basal metabolism is affected by age, size, body composition (muscle:fat ratios), and gender;[7] however, among people who are matched for these characteristics, basal metabolism varies at least 15 percent to either side of the mean.[8] In other words, people often have very slow or fast metabolisms for no apparent reason. These metabolic differences, of course, cause differences in the amount of food that will maintain body weight. In fact, researchers have studied pairs who have been matched for weight, height, age, sex, and activity level, where one of them habitually ate *twice* as much as the other.[9]

People's metabolic responses to eating and starving also vary. For instance, thin people's metabolisms tend to rise more than obese people's in response to sugar.[10] When thin people eat a lot, their bodies "rev up their engines" and burn extra energy, while obese people's bodies do so to a lesser extent. Obese people consistently gain at least twice as much as lean people when they are overfed the same amounts.[11]

Obese people also exhibit relatively large metabolic *decreases* in response to low-calorie diets. In other words, their bodies adjust to starvation more successfully and thereby keep them from losing as much weight.[12] These metabolic differences seem to be inborn; however, it is possible that long-term, frequent dieting increases the body's ability to conserve energy (and thereby preserve body fat) in response to low calorie intake.[13] Furthermore, it is likely that many chronic dieters are attempting to attain and maintain a weight that is too low (according to their body's standards), and consequently their bodies are responding with all the usual defense mechanisms of a person who is *underweight*. (More on this under Faulty Assumption #3.)

Faulty Assumption #3:
Each Person Needs a Certain
Number of Calories to Maintain Her
Weight; ±3,500 Calories = ±1 Pound

We also assume that only a certain number of calories will maintain our weight. In theory, we believe that this exact number can be specified. Many authors and doctors suggest formulas for estimating daily caloric need. For example, sedentary adults might be taught to multiply their weight times 15. Thus, an adult who weighs 130 would estimate her daily caloric need: $15 \times 130 = 1,950$ calories per day. Of course, we all know that activity levels vary from day to day, and that any estimate is rough. Nonetheless, the underlying principle remains: each day we need a certain number of calories—depending on our size, sex, activity level, age, etc.—and all deficits will cause body fat to be burned for energy, while all excess calories will be stored as fat.

Have you ever read in a diet book or heard from a doctor a mathematical explanation of the energy balance? If so, you have probably been told (and believed) that 3,500 calories equals one pound of body fat. In other words, if you eat 3,500 calories more than you need to maintain your weight, you expect to gain one pound. If you eat 3,500 calories less than you need, you expect to lose one pound. This is our third faulty assumption.

Experiments have shown that 3,500 "too few" or "too many" calories rarely result in the loss or gain of one pound. One study that examined controlled overfeeding of average-weight men found that the 3,500-calories-per-pound formula overestimated weight gain by more than half.[14] The men seemed to "burn off" a large portion of the excess calories automatically, and without increasing exercise levels. Furthermore, the heavier the men became, the less weight they gained on the same excessive diet.

Many skinny people—most often young men who have been taught that they should be "big and strong"—complain that they "can't gain weight." My first roommate was one of the few women I've known with the same problem. She often stuffed herself in order to gain weight, but it never worked. Her weight increases were, at best, fleeting. She did not gain one pound for every extra 3,500 calories she consumed—far from it.

The 3,500-calories-per-pound formula does little better in predicting weight loss. Obese people who decrease their caloric intake from 2,000 to 1,500 calories per day can expect to lose half as many pounds each month until the fourth month, when weight loss will approach or reach *zero*.[15] This is due to the body's automatic efforts to conserve energy in the face of starvation: the longer the deprivation, the more successfully the body conserves energy. If the food shortage is within a manageable range, the body will soon complete its adjustments and no longer need to burn fat for energy. Thus, what starts out as a "weight-loss diet" soon becomes a "maintenance diet."

Evidence also indicates that the longer people stay on low-calorie diets, the longer it takes for their metabolisms to return to normal.[16] Thus, dieting predisposes people to rapid weight gain immediately following the restrictions, and the longer the restrictions are maintained, the longer people will be predisposed to gain. Evidence also indicates that when people lose weight, they lose fat *and* protein, but when they regain, they regain mostly fat. Furthermore, when weight is lost, fat cells shrink, but when weight is gained, fat cells can *multiply*. These "fattening" effects of weight loss followed by weight gain are referred to as "overcompensation," which is apparently triggered by the loss of 20 percent or more of body weight. Some people seem to be protected from overcompensation by heredity. However, for everyone else, the result of overcompensation is that *repeated weight-loss dieting leads to higher and higher weights—the exact opposite of its purpose*.[17]

We can therefore understand the dieter's struggle in the following way. The longer she remains on the same low-calorie diet, the less weight she will lose (per week or month). The longer she maintains the diet and the more weight she loses, the longer her "rapid weight-gain phase" will last and the more weight she will regain. The more she weight-loss diets (followed by weight regain), the fatter she is likely to become.

Most dieters have had experiences that confirm these findings; but very few have been told that their difficulties are caused by automatic physiological defenses that oppose their efforts. They are not told that their caloric consumption will have to be repeatedly decreased in order to continue losing weight. They are not told that the amount of food which would have maintained their weights prior to a weight-loss diet will cause rapid weight gain after they lose weight. Because those who help people lose weight either do not know these things or fail to tell their clients, dieters are often left to blame themselves when they do not attain (or maintain) their goal weight. One woman told me that she had begun to fear that she ate in her sleep, as she could find no other explanation for her small weight losses and unexpected weight increases. Her doctor inspired this fear, in part, by refusing to believe that she ate as little as she reported. (He probably based his disbelief on the faulty 3,500-calorie-per-pound formula.)

In short, it is not true that only a certain number of calories will maintain a person's weight, nor is it true that 3,500 calories above or below this mythological number result in one-pound gains or losses. The physiology of weight loss and gain is far more complex than most people (including most weight-loss professionals and doctors) realize.

Faulty Assumption #4: Being Fat Is Unhealthy

How many times have you heard that the number one health hazard among Americans is overweight caused by overeating and lack of exercise? In 1959, the Metropolitan Life Insurance Company conducted a longevity and body weight study among its policyholders and reported that weights above certain ranges (according to height and sex) could be used to predict shorter life spans. Other sources informed us that obesity often causes high blood pressure, hypertension, and heart disease. In 1985, the National Institutes of Health Consensus Development Conference called obesity a "killer disease" and recommended weight loss to the thirty-four million Americans who exceed insurance standards by 20 percent or more.[18] Thus, the message has been loud and clear: excess weight is hazardous to health; allowing ourselves to be fat is self-destructive behavior; fat people will be healthier and live longer if they reduce. These assertions make up our fifth faulty assumption.

The relationship between weight and health is, at best, very difficult to pin down. In fact, statements such as "Being fat is unhealthy" or "Being thin is unhealthy" are completely *absurd* because they ignore the complexity of human beings and all the factors that affect health and longevity. Such statements also ignore the fact that scientific evidence currently points in conflicting directions when it comes to weight and health.

For instance, many researchers have reported correlations between certain health problems and high weight. However, high weight also correlates with a *lower incidence* of cancer, some respiratory diseases, many infectious diseases, osteoporosis (bone disease), some cardiovascular diseases, some gynecological and obstetric problems, anemia, diabetes type I, peptic ulcers, scoliosis, and suicide. In addition, obesity is associated with a more favorable prognosis in diabetes type II, hypertension, hyperlipemia, and rheumatoid arthritis.[19]

"But doesn't overweight cause premature death?" many would ask. Overall, research indicates it doesn't. Virtually every carefully controlled study, conducted both in and out of the United States, indicates that those who are significantly "overweight" (according to the current weight/height charts), but not "obese," have the *best* chance of surviving to old age, while those who are "model thin" (i.e., somewhat underweight) have the *least* chance of surviving to old age. More surprising still, there is evidence that even the so-called "morbidly obese" have a greater chance of surviving to old age than model-thin women![20]

But let's pause for a minute and ask, "What are all of these assertions based upon?" Answer: they are based upon *correlations*—in the last example, correlations between weight and death. And when dealing with correlations, it is important to remember the first commandment in statistical analysis, which is: correlation does not prove causation. In other words, two things can tend to happen at the same time without one *causing* the other.

For example, heart disease is more common among bald men,[21] so baldness *correlates* with heart disease. But that doesn't mean that baldness *causes* heart disease.

Clearly, it doesn't. The correlation is due to something other than direct cause and effect.

Another example: hypertension is more common among obese people,[22] so obesity correlates with hypertension. But does obesity cause hypertension? Probably not. In fact, recent research indicates that cycles of weight loss followed by weight gain may be causing hypertension among the obese, rather than "excess weight" per se.[23] This could explain why obese Samoan women rarely suffer from hypertension: they do not try to lose weight, therefore they do not harm their health with cycles of weight loss and gain.[24]

A final example: it is well documented that heavy people are prone to cardiovascular disorders. However, most studies fail to differentiate between people who are heavy owing in part to lots of muscle and people who are heavy owing primarily to lots of fat. Studies which examine this variable indicate that *excess muscle is the primary risk factor* for cardiovascular disorders. Those at greatest risk are muscular, have a large frame, and carry fat predominantly in the abdomen.[25] Thus, high weight correlates with cardiovascular disorders, but high weight does not cause these disorders. The functioning of the human body is far too complex for such a simplistic interpretation.

It is probably safe to assume that most correlations are due to something other than simple cause and effect. Nonetheless, correlations are constantly used to "prove" that one thing causes another. In the case of our culture's assumptions about weight and health, at least two mistakes have been made. First, assertions that being fat is unhealthy have been widely publicized, while literally hundreds of studies with results to the contrary have been ignored.[26] Second, we have been too quick to assume that being fat *causes* every health problem with which it correlates.

Space does not allow for an analysis of the hundreds of studies regarding weight and health that have been conducted to date. However, such an analysis is now available in *Rethinking Obesity* by Dr. Paul Ernsberger and Dr. Paul Haskew (see Resources, p. 240). The above discussion draws heavily from their research, but does not begin to cover it.

Most doctors are not up-to-date with current research on weight and health. Like the general public, they tend to be aware of the most widely publicized research, which is heavily biased against fatness. Because of this bias, a lot of very questionable, if not downright harmful, advice is being given on a regular basis.

I urge anyone who cares about this issue and *all of you* who have been told by a doctor or other health professional that you have a "weight problem" to get a copy of *Rethinking Obesity*, read the parts that interest you, and then, most important, *give it to your doctor*. If your doctor brushes you off with a claim of "being abreast of the literature," try to insist. Unless a doctor has spent an enormous amount of time and energy on this one subject, he or she will not have been able to keep abreast. In the case of doctors who have accepted the conclusions of the 1985 NIH Conference, it is essential that they read this book. The crucial issue is that you find a health care provider who is concerned enough to listen to you and to learn from current research.

In conclusion, it is extremely misleading, if not plain wrong, to say that being fat is unhealthy. Being fat increases the risk of some health problems and decreases the risk of others. Furthermore, starving an "endomorphic" (fat) person down to a lower weight does not magically change that person into an "ectomorph" (thin person). Fat and thin people are metabolically and genetically different from one another, and no amount of starving or force-feeding is going to change that. It is foolish to tell a thin person to force-feed herself to lower her risk of getting cancer, just as it is foolish to tell a fat person to starve herself to lower her risk of getting high blood pressure. *All* people can lower their health risks through good nutrition and regular exercise, but this will not change the fact that people come in all shapes and sizes —including big and fat. Luckily, most evidence indicates that this, in itself, is not a significant health problem.

Faulty Assumption #5: Fatness Is Caused by Life-Style, Not Heredity

Since we assume that fat people eat more than thin people and we blame people for how fat they are, it is not surprising that we also assume that body weight is not an inherited trait. Most people believe that fat parents tend to have fat children because they teach their children to eat too much and exercise too little. This is our fifth faulty assumption.

Researchers have known that body weight runs in families for over a century. As early as 1870 a French physician reported that most of his obese patients had at least one obese parent.[27] Modern studies have further shown that if one parent is fat, his or her child has a 50 percent chance of being fat, and when both parents are fat, their child has an 80 percent chance of being fat.[28]

Most people believe that fat parents teach children their own poor, excessive eating habits and sedentary life-styles. Although this sounds logical, evidence indicates that fatness is inherited much like other physical characteristics. We have already seen that fat people don't generally eat more than thin people. Therefore, it's ludicrous to claim that fat parents produce fat children by teaching them to be gluttons. Furthermore, we know that most fat people are metabolically different from most thin people, and it is equally ludicrous to claim that fat parents pass on their metabolic characteristics through upbringing.

One of the best ways to test this kind of nature/nurture controversy is through studies of twins. We can compare genetically identical twins to nonidentical twins. If amounts of body fat vary more among nonidentical than among identical twins, then it is probably due to genetic factors. Just such a study showed that the body weights of nonidentical twins were two and a half times more variable than the weights of identical twins. Furthermore, weights of nonidentical twins varied as much as weights of other, nontwin siblings.[29] Thus, identical twins have more similar body weights than nonidentical twins at least partly because genes determine body weight.

Another study compared identical twins who were raised in different environments. If upbringing and other environmental factors cause weight differences, we would expect many of the identical twins who grew up in different places to develop different eating habits, different life-styles, and, therefore, different weights. Most of the pairs showed differences in weight of five pounds or less. Five pairs showed larger differences in weight, but in all five cases chronic ill health (tuberculosis, for example) caused the differences.

One pair of identical twins was especially interesting. They were brought up in completely different types of environments and lived very differently. One lived on a farm, the other in a city; one contracted a serious disease (goiter), while the other did not; one married at seventeen and divorced at twenty-seven, while the other married at thirty-four and led a "placid married life." Nonetheless, at fifty-nine years of age, they weighed 208 and 221 pounds.

In short, inheritance has a powerful influence on body fat. Human beings come in many shapes and sizes, and genes determine, in part, each person's size and shape.

Faulty Assumption #6: Anyone Can Become and Remain Thin Through a "Sensible" Diet

Assumptions #1–#5 naturally lead to the belief that anyone can become and remain thin through a "sensible" and "healthy" diet. This is our sixth and final faulty assumption.

We have seen that fatness is due, to a large extent, to heredity and metabolism. Furthermore, low-calorie diets trigger physical reactions that oppose weight loss and may even promote escalating weight. Thus, it is clear that not everyone is capable of becoming and remaining thin through a "sensible" diet. In fact, advising chronically fat people to become thin is often the same as advising thin people to become and remain emaciated. They would have to function on a semistarvation diet and suffer from chronic feelings of hunger, tension, and tiredness; this would be neither "sensible" nor healthy.

This is not to say that it is impossible to lose weight through dietary changes. In fact, most Americans could lose *some* weight by improving the quality of their food intake. However, even if everyone ate in a healthy way, many people would still be fat, and most women would still be heavier than "model thin."

During my senior year of college, I exercised obsessively and ate the same things most of the time: one cup of shredded wheat with skim milk for breakfast; half a pita bread with low-fat cottage cheese and shredded cabbage for lunch; and steamed vegetables, a piece of boiled chicken (without skin), and sometimes a little brown rice for dinner. I wasn't dying of starvation, but I wasn't eating enough to be healthy and happy either. I was very underweight, and I suffered accordingly. I have known women who ate just as little in order to be of average weight for their height. They, too, suffered from the side effects of being underfed and underweight, but since they looked healthy, they assumed that their diet was "sensible" no matter how much pain it caused them.

Many chronic dieters skip breakfast alto-gether, eat a yogurt or salad for lunch, follow it up with a small dinner, and try to avoid other food by drinking large amounts of coffee or diet soda. Sound familiar? Some people may see this as a "sensible" form of weight control, but the price is food preoccupation and other unpleasant side effects. It's neither sensible nor healthy, whether it leads to emaciation, slenderness, an average weight, or an above-average weight.

These Faulty Assumptions Are Hazardous to Your Health and Happiness

Even though evidence contradicts these six faulty assumptions, they are extremely difficult to dislodge from people's minds. I have spent countless hours refuting each one for my friends and co-workers, only to find that although they agree with me by the end of the discussion, they continue to say and do things that are based on these assumptions. These people are not stupid or stubborn. Rather, they are constantly being brainwashed to accept the faulty assumptions. You, too, are under this insidious pressure. You see charts that list supposedly "healthy weights." You see magazine headlines promising tremendous weight losses with simple diets. Your family and friends may urge you to lose weight. All of it is based on the faulty assumptions refuted above. BE-WARE: even if you are *not* physically predisposed to being fat, these faulty assumptions are hazardous to your mental and physical well-being.

YOUR TRUE IDEAL WEIGHT: SETPOINT

You may be thinking, "This lady is crazy! She thinks that we should all be fat and proud of it!" Actually, that's not what I'm advocating. It can sound that way while I contradict myths about fatness, but I'm saying something different. Some of us are meant to be very thin; some of us are meant to be very fat; and most of us are meant to be somewhere in between. We all deserve to be at peace with our bodies instead of in a constant state of tension and dissatisfaction. We all deserve to be proud of ourselves and our bodies no matter how fat or thin we are.

How can we make peace with our bodies? Ultimately, we have to stop going on weight-loss diets. All of us can be healthier and happier if we stop battling with our bodies and accept a weight range that is *physiologically* appropriate. People come in all kinds of beautiful shapes and sizes! It is time that we celebrate that variety and drop the pressure to conform to one narrow image.

I have been recommending this viewpoint long enough to know that my opinions make people uncomfortable, and that only an extremely persuasive argument will override their deeply imbedded training. That's why I have carefully refuted many faulty assumptions about diet and weight. The next step is

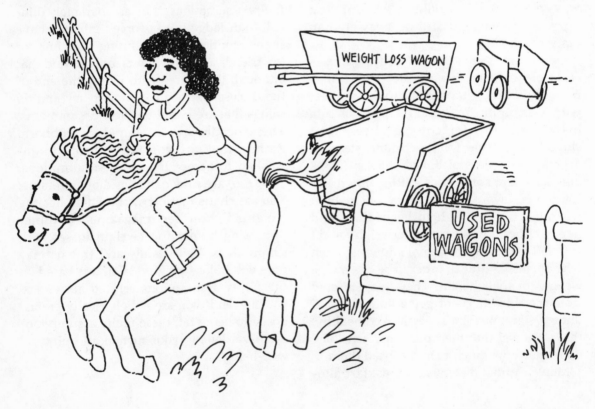

to replace those assumptions with a new understanding of weight maintenance, loss, and gain.

"Setpoint theory" explains the body's resistance to weight alteration better than any other theory to date. We have seen that low-calorie diets cause metabolic decreases, while overfeeding causes metabolic increases. These are examples of the body's attempts to defend its "setpoint" weight, the weight that is physiologically optimal. This physiologically optimal weight may or may not be within our culture's definition of what is "beautiful" or "normal."

Setpoint theory, then, proposes that "underweight" and "overweight" should be understood in terms of being above or below an individual's *setpoint weight*. A very thin woman may appear underweight but actually be at an appropriate weight for her body because she has an unusually low setpoint. Likewise, a very fat woman may appear overweight but actually be at (or even below) her setpoint. In general, we cannot see whether people are overweight or underweight because we cannot determine their setpoint weights just by looking.

What happens when people become underweight? Experimentally underfed people consistently experience serious side effects, including lower pulse, lower energy level, apathy, dizziness, intolerance to cold, slower metabolism (so that less food causes weight gain), a general preoccupation with food, intense hunger and cravings, a liking for previously disliked foods, lack of table manners, decreased sex drive, general irritability, and depression.[30]

Underfeeding causes physical and emo-tional hell as well as weight loss. In the study cited above,[30] participants were screened for emotional stability, and all began the experiment in high spirits. However, as the participants lost weight, they became increasingly irritable, depressed, and preoccupied with food. After about three months of underfeeding, their hunger became so intense that they felt unable to guarantee that they would control themselves away from the experimental site. A buddy system was developed to prevent cheating. Before the six-month experiment was over, two people suffered emotional breakdowns. Another subject cut off the end of a finger, apparently hoping that he would be excused from the study. In short, the participants found the side effects of underfeeding and underweight *intolerable*.

These severe problems persisted several months after the food restrictions ended. Several of the participants ate as many as *11,000 calories in a day* but complained that they still felt hungry. Thus being underweight causes feelings of insatiability: even very large meals fail to satisfy.

We know that the side effects of underfeeding and underweight are natural and virtually inevitable. Chronic dieters readily recognize themselves in that long list of side effects. Their experiences are similar because when they limit their eating and lose weight, they are actually becoming underfed and underweight (even though they may not look it).

A study of obese people's responses to weight loss supported this theory: researchers observed physical and emotional side effects like those of thin people who were underfed. The participants did not become like average-weight people by losing weight.[31]

Dr. Hilde Bruch's observations of people who suffer from eating disorders also supports setpoint theory. She asserts that if an individual's weight is stable and her eating patterns are reasonably comfortable, then attempts to reduce are inadvisable unless a specific health problem demands it. She has repeatedly observed that although some fat people initially lose weight, they are healthier and happier at the higher, more stable weight. She concludes that these higher weights are physiologically and psychologically optimal, while weights chosen according to a standard weight chart, or cultural ideas of "beauty," are inappropriate and harmful.

Bruch further supports this view in her discussion of "fat-thin" people. She observes that many people who lose weight and maintain slim figures do so only via semistarvation diets that cause continuous strain, tension, and ill health.[32] Thus, it is *possible* to force one's body below its setpoint, but only at tremendous mental and physical cost.

I interviewed competitive wrestlers and rowers whose experiences support setpoint theory in yet another way. All the athletes reported stable off-season weights and relaxed eating patterns; however, during their athletic seasons, while they were forced to attain lower weights, their eating patterns and feelings toward food were similar to those of people who have eating disorders.

All the athletes said that although they knew they should lose weight gradually and then maintain the losses, with the exception of one rower, they *never* managed to do it that way. Many had repeatedly promised themselves that they would "do it right" next season, but then found that they could not keep their vows. Sound familiar? How many dieters do you know with the same problem?

Instead, the athletes reduced their weights to within ten to twenty pounds of their target weights and yo-yoed up and down every week. These weight swings were caused by alternating between very limited diets (or fasts), with little liquid intake, and binges. Each week they ate huge amounts of food the day or two after they "made weight" (athlete's slang for achieving their required weights prior to competitions) and then starved themselves throughout the remainder of the week in order to make weight for the next competition.

A few athletes also made themselves vomit in order to avoid gaining weight and relieve pain caused by overeating. *All* the athletes shared a weekly practice of eating until in pain. They explained that these binges were caused by *insatiable hunger* (hunger that persists despite eating). They also said they felt "entitled" to eat as much as they wanted after competitions to relieve the unbearable tension and self-deprivation of the previous days.

Not only did the athletes binge on a weekly basis, they binged very frequently for the first two to six weeks after the season ended. One wrestler stated, "I always promise myself that I won't eat too much at the end of the season, but then I lose control. I just *have* to have something every minute."

Another wrestler's experiences paralleled his wrestling peers' in every way but one: he looked "normal" at his wrestling weight and looked "heavy" off-season. (All other wrestlers were extremely thin at their wrestling weights.) He stated that during his worst moments people told him that he looked great; however, he knew that he was "miserable, irritable, starved, very underweight . . . and therefore couldn't possibly enjoy life at that weight." The fact that this man experienced all the same physical and psychological problems associated with underfeeding and underweight suggests that he had a setpoint weight that was higher—demanded more body fat—than the other wrestlers'.

The athletes' descriptions of insatiability, painful bingeing, and purging are almost exactly like those of people who suffer from chronic dieting and bulimia. The one important difference is that the athletes see their insatiability and bingeing as normal and inevitable reactions to their seasonal starvation and weight loss. Since they don't have eating or weight problems when they maintain higher weights off-season, the causes of their playing-season misery are obvious. They may promise themselves to resist the desire to overeat for the first few seasons; however, they soon learn that *it is virtually impossible to avoid bingeing unless they avoid starving and cutting weight.* If they can't stand the agony of cutting weight, then they have to give up competitive wrestling or rowing. If wrestling or rowing is very important to them, then they resign themselves to the yearly starvation and the inevitable result: physical pain and emotional instability.

Chronic dieters, on the other hand, tend to assume that their discomfort and feelings of insatiability are due to *psychological* problems. They, too, promise themselves to resist the desire to overeat. But when they experience the profound effects of undereating, they blame their behavior on psychological problems and a lack of self-discipline. The truth is that such behavior is a virtually inevitable result of self-starvation and weight loss. Since their attempts to lose weight are inspired by inflexible concepts of "beauty," rather than seasonal sports, they don't see a light at the end of the tunnel. They can't look forward to the "end of the season," nor do they see the option of giving up the "sport."

Is this hitting close to home? Your "sport" is the pursuit of slenderness for the sake of "beauty." You probably want to be thinner than your body was designed to be, and so you have tried to starve or purge yourself down to size. We know what happens when people starve themselves and fall below their setpoints: they suffer so horribly that even previously well-adjusted people sometimes have nervous breakdowns. Your preoccupation with diet and weight (hunger, bingeing, cravings, depression, etc.) probably isn't caused by "psychological problems"—it's all part of the sport.

Refining Setpoint Theory

We must beware of oversimplifying setpoint theory. People sometimes get the idea that "setpoint" refers to *one* weight that our bodies are physiologically programmed to defend no matter what we do. Setpoint theory is a little more complex than that. Setpoint weights are the result of both genetic influence *and* diet/life-style; therefore, our setpoint weights change when our diets and life-styles change.

Regular aerobic exercise promotes a lower setpoint. This is different from saying that if we exercise we will burn more calories and lose weight. The number of additional calories we burn through, for instance, half an hour of jogging or rapid swimming (rather than a sedentary activity) are insignificant. The food equivalents are laughable. Therefore, if exercise simply burned a few extra calories during workouts, then exercise would have little impact on weight.[33]

If, on the other hand, exercise lowers setpoint weight, then our bodies respond to regular exercise by metabolically (and otherwise) defending a lower weight. This theory is supported by the experiences of people who try to lose weight. Exercise can help them lose weight, but maintaining the losses without maintaining the exercise programs is extremely difficult.

Diets high in simple sugars, refined carbohydrates (e.g., white flour), and fats seem to promote relatively high setpoint weights.[34] This means that when we eat only low-fat, low-sugar foods and replace refined carbohydrates with whole grains, our bodies automatically try to maintain a lower weight than when we eat like most Americans. This is different from claiming that if we *eat less* we will lose weight. We are talking about a change in *quality*, not *quantity*. If a change in quality alone lowers setpoint weight, then we can eat as much as we want yet automatically maintain a lower weight.

Setpoint theory is a new conceptualization of the way our bodies gain and lose weight. It proposes that our bodies have an invested interest in our body fat: we are most comfortable with a certain amount of fat. This amount depends on genetic factors, diet, and levels of exercise. Thus a woman may have a setpoint weight of 190 pounds when she is inactive and eats like most Americans; her setpoint may drop to 178 if she eliminates sugar and drastically reduces the fat content of her diet; and her setpoint might be 166 if she also begins to exercise on a regular basis. By comparison, a woman of the same height could have a setpoint of 130 when she is inactive and eats like most Americans, and be able to lower her setpoint from there (though in much smaller amounts) through exercise and diet. (These numbers are used to illustrate a point rather than to indicate how many pounds the setpoints are likely to move.) The point is: although life-style affects weight, we *inherit* our setpoint weight ranges.

Setpoint theory allows for the fact that we can change our weight permanently through permanent changes in diet and life-style; however, it also maintains that some people are genetically designed to be fatter than others. Those who attempt to reduce their weights by eating less (rather than changing the types of food they eat and/or their activity level) will be likely to reduce their weights without reducing their setpoints, and will therefore be underweight according to their bodies' standards, suffer accordingly, and regain weight very easily.

Many people who are preoccupied with diet and weight have chosen a "goal weight" that lies outside their setpoint weight ranges altogether. In other words, they have chosen a weight that is considered attractive but that can never be healthy or comfortable for them regardless of life-style and food choices. They continue to struggle toward their misguided goal, not knowing that they cannot reach it without becoming underfed and underweight and suffering accordingly. BEWARE: you, too, may have chosen an inappropriate goal weight.

Setpoint and Aging

How does age affect setpoint weight? In general, setpoints rise with age. Evidence indicates that how much they rise is heavily influenced by body type.

Body types can be classified as primarily ectomorphic (light boned and thin), mesomorphic (muscular), or endomorphic (fat). (This is an oversimplification but will suffice for our purposes.) William Sheldon and his colleagues tracked weight and age over twenty years and found that body type predicts changes in weight. In general, ectomorphs gain little weight with age despite hearty eating, while endomorphs and some mesomorphs gain considerably despite normal caloric intake. Thus, it seems that an increase in weight with age is natural for some and not for others.

Age-specific studies of mortality and weight indicate that those who gain weight with age more often survive into old age than those who do not gain weight. In response to these findings, Reubin Andres has recommended age-specific height-weight tables that allow for a gain of approximately one pound per year from age thirty to seventy.[35]

Thus, the common assumption that one should weigh the same at age fifty as one weighed at twenty-five is probably misguided. It may be healthy and natural for many ectomorphs to weigh close to the same weight over their lifetimes; however, most people naturally gain weight with age, and evidence indicates that *not* allowing this natural gain to occur increases one's chances for an early grave.

Why We Crave

Do you ever crave specific foods, or specific types of food? Have you ever felt that your yearning for sweets was excessive and abnormal? Your cravings are not just in your mind. They often have physical causes.

We have already seen that being underweight causes insatiability. Studies also indicate that being underweight, or having an unstable weight, causes an "extended taste responsiveness" to sugar. When "normal," stable-weight people consume a certain amount of a sweet drink, they lose their taste for it. People who are underweight continue to enjoy it. This is one of the body's mechanisms for encouraging increased consumption and weight gain in response to weight loss. One study compared the taste responsiveness of "static" obese people (weights stable for two years or more) and "dynamic" obese people (weights unstable from repeated dieting). Most static obese people responded to sweet solution as "normal" weight people do, while dynamic obese people responded like underweight people.[36]

What does this mean? First, if extended taste responsiveness is a symptom of being underweight, then it again seems that most obese people have higher setpoints than we recognize as legitimate "ideal weights." This evidence also helps explain sweet-food binges, which are common among chronic dieters and bulimics. Long binges on sweet foods tend to be very unpleasant for people who are at stable, appropriate (setpoint) weights. After a while the food tastes "sickeningly sweet" and is no longer desirable. People who chronically diet or are below their setpoint weights, on the other hand, may enjoy a long binge on sweet food because they do not lose their taste for it: their bodies are crying out for the calories. If this is true, then people who binge on sweets will be less likely to do so if they maintain a comfortable (setpoint) weight because they will lose their extended taste responsiveness.

Studies also indicate that cravings for other foods, such as carbohydrates (starches), can have a physiological basis. Diets even moderately high in protein (over 10 percent of calories) increase carbohydrate appetite.[37] The average American consumes well over this amount of protein (estimates vary from 12 to 18 percent), and most weight-loss diets are even higher in protein. Some fad diets exceed 50 percent protein. Thus, most weight-loss diets, as well as the average American diet, probably lead to physiologically induced carbohydrate cravings.

Dieters often report that evenings and periods of emotional and physical stress bring on the most intense carbohydrate cravings. This, too, may be explained physiologically. Eating carbohydrates triggers the release of a special chemical in the brain called serotonin. Serotonin suppresses the desire for more carbohydrates, induces sleepiness, and decreases sensitivity to pain.[38] Therefore, the relief people experience from eating carbohydrates at night and during stressful times is (at least partly) physiologically induced. *Psychological* explanations for carbohydrate cravings are often misguided.

These findings have important implications for people who are preoccupied with diet and weight. Most of you have tried to limit carbohydrate intake because you have been taught that bread, potatoes, rice, and similar foods are low in nutrients and high in calories. (This is a myth: *complex* carbohydrates are neither particularly high in calories nor particularly low in nutritional value.) Most of you have also been encouraged to believe that cravings are "neurotic" symptoms that you should overcome. Consequently, when you eat in response to cravings, you probably feel guilty and annoyed. If you avoid carbohydrates, then of course you crave them—that is your body expressing its needs. If you starve yourself, then of course you crave high-calorie foods—that, too, is your body expressing its needs. We all have a lot to learn from our own bodies. They know more about our needs than a lot of the "experts" who tell us otherwise.

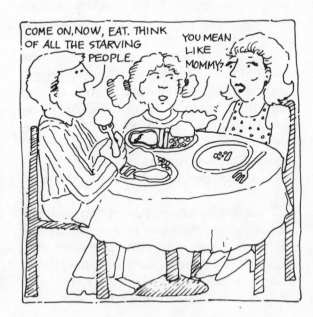

YOUR BODY AND DIET/WEIGHT CONFLICT

We now know that you have a setpoint weight that your body is attempting to defend with strong physiological mechanisms. If you try to override your setpoint through weight-loss diets, an unhealthy and painful battle between your body and yourself is inevitable. Your body will adjust to lower caloric intake through lower metabolic rates. And once you fall below your setpoint, you may experience insatiability, food preoccupation, strong cravings, extended taste responsiveness, decreased energy levels, apathy, decreased sexual urges and responsiveness, amenorrhea (lack of periods), increased sensitivity to cold, general irritability, and inexplicable depression.

Most of us believe that if we are unable to control our diet and weight, it is due to personal weaknesses and psychological problems. We repeatedly try to override and control our hunger in order to attain and maintain lower weights. Our bodies try to force us to give ourselves what we want and need (more food!); and we try to force our bodies to "make do," continue to function, and give up our body fat. We wage a war with our own bodies.

I hope that this chapter has led you to consider that attempts to lose weight may be causing a battle between you and your body. The pursuit of slenderness very often leads to diet/weight preoccupation and eating disorders resulting from *physiological* responses to dieting and weight loss. Regardless of your present size, and regardless of why you pursue slenderness, the source of your preoccupation is not "all in your mind." Your body is deeply involved in the struggle.

PERSONAL QUESTIONS:
ESTIMATING YOUR SETPOINT WEIGHT RANGE

Most people finish this chapter with a burning and terrifying question: "What is my setpoint weight range?" This is a difficult question to answer. If you have been suffering from diet and weight conflicts since *before* you were full grown, it is especially hard to answer.

Luckily, you don't need to know your setpoint weight in order to work toward, and attain, freedom from diet/weight preoccupation. The personal process you must go through to attain this freedom is the same regardless of your setpoint weight; in fact, the key to overcoming your preoccupation is to *stop thinking about pounds and thinness*, which means that it might be better if you never gave weight (setpoint or otherwise) another thought.

Why, then, am I going to help you determine your setpoint range? First, because I know that if I don't, you will try to determine (or imagine) it anyway. Second, because some of you will find accurate information about your body liberating.

How can this be liberating? When I was in college, I obtained medical records that documented my height and weight before and during adolescence. The numbers I saw shocked me. I knew that I was underweight at 97 pounds, but I had no idea *how* underweight. The medical records revealed that at fifteen years of age, before I developed a diet/weight problem and before I was physically mature, I weighed 110 pounds.

I was very slender, and well aware of it, when I was fifteen. I was healthy, I exercised regularly, and I ate freely and noncompulsively. When I learned that 110 pounds had been an appropriate weight for me as a flat-chested fifteen-year-old, it became obvious that my adult setpoint weight was *over* 110!

This knowledge was liberating because it forced me to acknowledge a more reasonable "ideal weight." I did not immediately want or try to gain weight, but I was able to change the way in which I *thought* about my weight. Learning to *feel* differently about my weight involved a much longer and more difficult process. However, it was the realization that I was struggling to be underweight that set the stage for my recovery from severe diet/weight conflict.

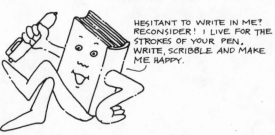

HESITANT TO WRITE IN ME?
RECONSIDER! I LIVE FOR THE
STROKES OF YOUR PEN.
WRITE, SCRIBBLE AND MAKE
ME HAPPY.

1.   Are either of your parents or any of your siblings fat and/or suffering from diet/weight conflict? If so, list their names here.

If there is a history of "weight problems" in your family, you are more likely to have a somewhat high setpoint weight. However, family history may tell you less than your own weight history. Therefore, get medical records (regarding height and weight) and list these and other weight fluctuations you can remember.

WEIGHT HISTORY

Age	Height	Weight	Activity Level	Restrictive Diets?

Ceasing to Diet and Discovering Our Setpoints

2. Did your diet/weight conflicts begin before or after you reached your adult height? If *after*, what was your highest weight prior to your concern about diet/weight?

3. Has your weight ever remained fairly *stable* while you were not dieting? If so, what was (were) the stable weight(s)?

These are important questions, because an adult weight that was reached and/or maintained *effortlessly* was probably within an appropriate weight range for your body and life-style at that time.

4. Is there a weight to which you tend to return after weight-loss diets? If so, what weight?

Weights to which you tend to return after diets, of course, are likely to be closer to your setpoint than are the weights to which you reduce. It may be, however, that these weights are higher than your setpoint because of your body's reactive and protective response to weight-loss dieting.

5. Have you ever gotten aerobic exercise on a regular basis (e.g., continuous brisk walking, running, swimming, or biking for twenty-five minutes or more, three or more times per week) over a long period of time? If so, how much was your weight affected?

6.   Have you ever gotten very little or no exercise for a long period of time? If so, how much was your weight affected?

Regular aerobic exercise usually lowers setpoint. If you have had significant changes in activity level over time, then you may be able to estimate the amount your setpoint changes as a result of exercise.

7.   Have you ever eaten mostly low-fat, low-sugar foods and whole grains rather than refined carbohydrates (e.g., whole wheat bread instead of white, brown rice instead of white) over a long period of time? If so, how much was your weight affected?

8.   Have you ever eaten a lot of high-fat, high-sugar foods and processed grains on a daily basis over a long period of time? If so, how much was your weight affected?

Dietary sugar, fat, and refined carbohydrates, when eaten on a regular basis, raise setpoint. If the *quality* of your food has changed significantly over time, you may be able to estimate the amount your setpoint changes as a result of the kinds of food you eat.

9.   Have you ever consumed a lot of stimulants, either by smoking, drinking a lot of coffee, or taking other drugs? If so, how much was your weight affected?

Large doses of stimulants usually lower setpoint. They are also addictive and physically harmful (particularly smoking). Therefore, it is a good idea to avoid or limit stimulants, yet be aware of the likely effect on setpoint.

10. Look at each item on the following list and check off all the problems you have experienced at any time since you began to struggle with diet and weight.

☐ getting cold easily

☐ tolerating heat easily

☐ exaggerated anticipation of eating

☐ cravings for specific foods or type s of food

☐ preoccupation with food

☐ feelings of desperate hunger

☐ decreased (or lack of) sexual desires/needs/responsiveness

☐ amenorrhea (loss of menstrual periods)

☐ increased apathy

☐ increased fatigue

☐ slowed activity (e.g., moving more slowly)

☐ increased irritability

☐ increased depression

☐ insatiability (can eat a lot and still feel hungry)

☐ extended taste responsiveness to sweet foods

11. How much have you weighed when these problems were at their worst?

The problems listed under question 10 are common symptoms of being underweight and/or underfed. Thus, if you can determine that at certain weights you experience many of these problems, then you should suspect that your setpoint weight is higher than those weights. (You could also experience some of these problems in response to weight-loss diets even when you are not underweight.)

MAKING PEACE WITH FOOD

12. Has your desired weight—the weight you want to achieve and maintain—changed since you were full grown? If so, in what direction and why?

If your desired weight has gone up, it is probably because: (a) you found the cost of maintaining an inappropriately low weight too unpleasant and have therefore begun to recognize/accept your body type, and/or (b) your setpoint has risen with age. If, on the other hand, your desired weight has become progressively lower, you are probably attempting to boost your self-esteem through weight loss and diet control. Meanwhile, your desired weight has been becoming less and less "desirable" for your physical and mental health. You need to reverse this trend.

13. In light of the information you have gathered, try to estimate your setpoint weight range:

Approximate Setpoint   *Accompanying Life-Style**

Setpoint Weight Range

_____ = very sedentary, very high fat/sugar/refined carbohydrate intake

_____ = little aerobic excercise, high fat/sugar/refined carbohydrate intake

_____ = little aerobic exercise, moderate fat/sugar/refined carbohydrate intake

_____ = aerobic exercise 3-4 times a week, moderate fat/sugar/refined carbohydrate intake

_____ = aerobic exercise 3-4 times a week, low fat/sugar/refined carbohydrate intake

_____ = fanatical exercise, very low fat, no sugar or refined carbohydrate intake

* Note that you could "mix and match" the variables that affect setpoint in many other ways. Except at the extreme ends of the spectrum, the life-styles described are a just few examples of the many permutations that could promote the different parts of your setpoint weight range.

Ceasing to Diet and Discovering Our Setpoints

14. Let's assume, for the sake of argument, that your setpoint weight is higher than you consider aesthetically ideal. List all the benefits you stand to gain from being as slim as your ideal versus the costs of maintaining that (under setpoint) weight.

BENEFITS OF UNDERWEIGHT	COSTS OF UNDERWEIGHT

15. Now make another benefit-versus-cost comparison, this time for accepting and maintaining this hypothetically high setpoint weight.

BENEFITS OF SETPOINT	COSTS OF SETPOINT

In all likelihood, this conflict between what you would like to weigh and your setpoint is not hypothetical. Most people, particularly those who are preoccupied with diet and weight, would like to be thinner than their bodies dictate. Therefore, you need to consider the benefits and costs of what, right now, feels like a choice between two "evils." It is a choice between: (a) trying to be thinner than your setpoint (and sometimes succeeding), remaining chronically preoccupied with diet and weight, and feeling physically uncomfortable, and (b) being heavier, recovering your ability to eat freely without preoccupation or guilt, and feeling well.

16.   At this moment, which seems to be the lesser of two evils for you: being heavier than you want to be or paying the mental and physical cost of being underweight?

If you answered the latter, or if you could not choose either one, do not blame yourself. You are not alone. Many of you are probably feeling panicky and depressed right now. You may be feeling doomed to a lifetime of struggle with food and weight, or a lifetime of being "fat" and unhappy. Try to relax and realize that you are not helpless. Remember that you always have options, and that you are never really "doomed" (unless nuclear bombs are being dropped). Right now you may feel as though you cannot be happy unless you're thin, or at least working toward that goal. Don't believe it! It's not true. Many of you are probably not ready to give up destructive goals and diets. That's okay. If you're not ready, then don't give them up. This is a complex process of change, contradicting all we've been taught about ourselves and our bodies. You needn't rush into anything. Set your own pace, and take one step at a time.

3

LEARNING TO LOVE
OUR BODIES

It was morning. I was still in bed. And for the first time since I had become a full-grown woman, I touched my rounded, protruding belly. And I thought, "I'm stroking me. I'm appreciating me." That part of my body that had long remained an alien structure, toward which I felt only hate, anger, and shame, became the center of my body and the center of myself. Herein lies a strong, beautiful, kind, creative, and intelligent woman. Herein lies a source of new life—here, right here, under my hand. I finally saw and felt that my curving fullness was beautiful. And then the hiding, and the sucking inward, and the flattening, pain, and shame ... seemed alien. I knew that I would no longer constrict or hide the center of my body and myself. I arose and began my celebration. I reached out to others saying, "Come celebrate with me."

THE AUTHOR'S DREAM

AESTHETIC IDEALS AND ORNAMENTAL BODY VIEWS

The first seed of our preoccupation is the thought "I'm too fat." Where this thought never appears, a preoccupation with diet and weight never develops. Unfortunately, this thought is extremely common, and we hear people voice it every day. Our society is overrun by people who think they're too fat. Since this is where our problem begins, we need to know why so many people share this view of their bodies.

One question I love to ask people who complain that they're too fat is "Too fat for what?" This question is usually considered absurd; hence, people usually respond by laughing or glaring at me. "Too fat to walk?" No. "Too fat to make love?" No. "Too fat to be fit?" No. "Too fat to swim or play tennis or run or cycle or hike or dance ...?" No, only rarely. This can go on for quite a while, but in the end the truth emerges: "Too fat to be 'attractive.' " It's an aesthetic judgment. The most common reason why people want to be thinner is that they think they will look better.

Long, thin bodies are constantly displayed, admired, and idealized all around us. As we walk down the street, we see emaciated female forms staring out at us from countless shop windows. They display designer jeans, leotards, dresses, bathing suits, underwear. . . . We end up thinking, "That's how I should look!"

On television we see thin adolescent models, made up like adults, doing advertisements for adult women's clothing. And we think that, too, is how we should look. Most actresses and adult models are equally thin (if they weren't, they would probably lose their jobs), and we look at them and ask ourselves: "If they can do it, why can't I?"

If we go to high school or college, we see and talk to hoards of young women who almost constantly diet, and worry and talk about their weight. If they are thin, they usually display their bodies in showy, tight clothing. And if they're not thin, they hide their bodies in loose clothing, avoid horizontal stripes, and try to lose weight.

This very thin "ideal" is inappropriate and unhealthy for nearly all of us. It is appropriate for a small group of people who have inherited a very lean and small-boned body type; however, most women do not fall into this category. Modeling agencies have been known to suggest that women who are five feet tall should weigh 100 pounds, and that for every inch of height over five feet, women should add 3 pounds. These aesthetically based recommendations are 2 to 3 pounds *below* the lowest recommended

weights listed in the current U.S. chart. Thus, according to current medical standards, the weights that aesthetic ideals prescribe are too low even for women with small frames.

Unfortunately, women choose their ideal weights with these aesthetic ideals in mind.[1] Consequently, women who are well within healthy weight ranges nonetheless consider themselves overweight and therefore try to reduce.[2] This destructive behavior is not surprising, given our environment. We are surrounded by advertisements for spas and clinics and special foods and books and pills and programs, all claiming they can help us get thinner. That we want to be thin and that we should be thin is assumed: everyone has learned that! The only question is: are we going to "go after it" and "be all that we can be," or are we too weak-willed and lazy to do so?

Most of us can hardly imagine a different set of aesthetic standards and attitudes because we are so deeply immersed in the prevailing madness. Everyone "knows" that a woman has to be lean to be beautiful—right? This is what I mean when I say that we are surrounded by "aesthetically thin minds": people who not only hold a very thin aesthetic ideal, but who are also very *narrow-minded* regarding what body types are attractive and acceptable.

You probably have an aesthetically thin mind, too. Within this culture it's difficult to think in any other way. However, in order to overcome your conflicts with diet and weight, you have got to develop a different perspective: a broader appreciation for the human body and its variety.

Many people have tried to convince me

that there is something "natural" about a preference for leanness and that we have an instinctual repugnance for fatness. The truth is that people learn their concept of beauty from the media and the people around them. Every society has its own aesthetic ideals—definitions of what's attractive and what's ugly, what's sexy and what's not. These ideals vary from culture to culture, and change over time. History suggests that whatever is more difficult to achieve, and is therefore more unusual, becomes idealized. Thus, when food is scarce, heavy figures are idealized; when food is abundant, slender figures are idealized.[3]

Most people's aesthetic preferences are reflections of the cultural ideals to which they are exposed. However, we can find exceptions to the rule. Beauty really is in the eye of the beholder. Even within our "fattist" culture, some people find fat bodies more attractive and sexy than thin bodies. In fact, some people have joined together to share their appreciation of fatness, and to support each other in the face of attitudes that make them feel like social outcasts.[4]

Those of us who idealize slenderness—but wish we didn't—can broaden our appreciation of the human body in a number of ways: we can join groups that are fat-appreciative and antifattist; if economically feasible, we can travel to countries where thin is not "in"; and we can look into history and try to develop our own love of fat bodies.

Imagine a society where, in films, fat women are idealized, admired, and loved, while hoards of slender women gaze at their physical abundance with envy (India is a contemporary example). Imagine a place and time where advertising and pornography focus on fat and/or pregnant women because they are considered the sexiest, most womanly, most sensual, and most beautiful. Many famous artists idealized full-figured women: Titian (real name: Tiziano Vecellio, about 1490–1576), Peter Paul Rubens (1577–1640), and Auguste Renoir (1841–1919), to name a few. All of these artists spent much of their time painting, etching, or sculpting women who are fat by today's standards.

Of course, I am not trying to say that fat aesthetic ideals are somehow "better" than thin aesthetic ideals. I would hate to see thin women feeling unattractive because they're thin, just as I now hate to see most women feeling unattractive because they're not "thin enough." Hilde Bruch quotes a French physician who, in 1911, wrote:

> One must mention here that aesthetic errors of a worldly nature to which all women submit, may make them want to stay obese for reasons of fashionable appearance. It is beyond a doubt that in order to have an impressive décolleté each woman feels herself duty bound to be fat around the neck, over the clavicle and in her breasts. Now it happens that fat accumulates with greatest difficulty in these places ... one cannot obtain weight reduction without ... the woman sacrificing in her spirits the upper part of her body. To her it is a true sacrifice because she gives up what the world considers beautiful.[5]

Thus, fat aesthetic ideals led to painful and unhealthy stuffing in 1911, while today's thin aesthetic ideals lead to painful and unhealthy starving. The harmful underlying belief is the same: we should conform to

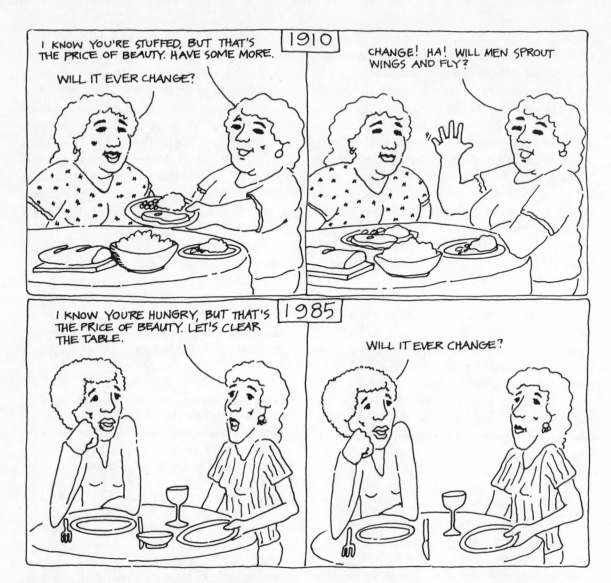

prevailing aesthetic ideals regardless of cost. It's time we throw out all of these exclusive "ideals," and say: "No—we will not take part in it! We can appreciate a wide range of human physiques, and we will not conform (and will support others who refuse to conform) to destructive societal 'ideals.'"

Not long ago a young chronic dieter and bulimic asked me what I thought of *The Obsession* by Kim Chernin. I told her that I found it very valuable, and she said, "While I was reading it, I began to think and feel that maybe my body wasn't so bad after all —that maybe I was okay just as I was. But then I had to stop myself because I knew it was just an excuse for not dieting."

MAKING PEACE WITH FOOD

Most of us, just like this young woman, are very well trained. When we begin to break away from destructive social norms, we are quickly pulled back: "Wait . . . I can't think this way. It's bad; it's an excuse; it's just a way of giving up." But if we find and create support for our efforts and realize that it's good and perfectly legitimate to love our bodies no matter how fat, thin, small, or gigantic we are, then we can hold on to those sweet, sane moments a bit longer, and a bit longer, and a bit longer . . . until finally we completely embrace those thoughts and feelings in our hearts and minds and never let them go.

Just as we can develop a broader appreciation of art or music, we can develop a broader appreciation of the human body. The cost of our aesthetically thin minds is very high, in terms of both the hell we suffer and the damage we do to others. Why accept such a narrow and harmful viewpoint when we can learn to appreciate and enjoy the beauty of larger, fatter bodies in addition to the beauty of thin and lean bodies?

To help us gain full appreciation for our bodies, we can also change our way of "seeing" them. Most people have been trained to judge people's bodies (especially women's bodies) *ornamentally:* is she attractive? Our society has a long history of judging women's bodies (and often the women themselves) *exclusively* on this basis.

Among a random sample of fifty college students, I found that general questions regarding body satisfaction led most women to talk about their appearance, while the same questions led most men to talk about their health and athletic ability. Women automatically judged their bodies on an ornamental basis, while men judged their bodies on an instrumental basis.

People should not feel that they must be "slender" and/or "athletic" in order to feel good about their bodies. However, we automatically want to be healthy and physically comfortable, because these promote well-being. If women judged their bodies instrumentally, many fewer women would feel "too fat." The very thin ideals women now pursue have no instrumental value. On the contrary, virtually every woman who continually struggles to maintain a slender ideal would be healthier, and no less able-bodied, if she stopped fighting with her body and accepted a higher weight. The amount of weight she would have to gain before any instrumentally negative effect took hold would be far beyond the point at which she would consider herself "fat."

In our society, women who are fifteen pounds over the national average consider themselves fat, while men do not define themselves as such until they are thirty-five pounds above average![6] Perhaps men tend to define themselves as fat when they begin to *feel* fat because of restricted movement or some other problem associated with their weight, while women define themselves as fat as soon as they "look fat."

Most women who struggle for the very thin thighs, modest hips, and completely flat bellies* our aesthetic ideals prescribe become

* People often claim that rounded abdomens are caused by a lack of stomach muscles, and anyone who builds stomach muscles will have a flat abdomen. This is simply untrue. Most women are meant to have rounded abdomens, and many can have muscle-bound stomachs and nevertheless have rounded abdomens. The pursuit of an unnaturally flat abdomen has lead countless women to lose more and more weight, always hoping that if they

Learning to Love Our Bodies

underweight and therefore experience many of the negative side effects discussed in Chapter 2. Why do so many intelligent people torture themselves in pursuit of slenderness? Why, even after they experience the high cost of this pursuit (chronic tension, hunger, insatiability, food preoccupation, sensitivity to cold), do they continue to torture themselves?

I have discussed four major reasons why women who suffer in this way rarely question the value of the aesthetic ideals they pursue: (a) they don't realize that their physical and psychological torment is at least partly caused by trying to be too thin; (b) the media, family members, friends, and acquaintances tell them that they can and *should* be thin; (c) they have been taught to view their bodies as ornaments rather than instruments through which to act and live; and (d) they feel an urgent, overriding desire and need to be "beautiful," as society defines it. Although it is easy to see that an ornamental body view leads to a strong desire to be beautiful, we still need to investigate specific examples of how our society "convinces" (conditions, socializes, brainwashes) a woman to view herself in this way. For it is only through extensive and continual conditioning that an intelligent human being comes to see herself as an ornament, whose first priority is the attainment of a slender body, rather than as a

complete human being who has a myriad of other concerns and unlimited potential.

THE OBJECTIFICATION OF WOMEN

Our society continually objectifies women, which leads most women to objectify themselves. It is important to understand what it means to "objectify," because objectification affects the way we think and feel about people, including ourselves. To objectify people is to look at them and treat them like objects —to focus solely on appearance. It is to externalize people—to ignore their intelligence, abilities, and feelings. Thus, when we objectify people, we dehumanize them.

Two of the purest forms of objectification are beauty contests and body-building contests. Beauty contestants are paraded across stages like so many units of flesh, bone, and fashion, and judged on purely aesthetic grounds. With the exception of token "talent" and "question" portions of the contests, they are glorified lessons in the practice of objectification. Body-building contests involve the same pure form of objectification, only the aesthetic ideal—the valued type of appearance—is different. In both cases, the audience objectifies the contestants, and the contestants objectify themselves and each other. Who they are, what they think, what they want, what they are capable of accomplishing . . . all of this is irrelevant. The important question is: do they look like they are "supposed to"? Their value is judged and compared according to one rigid image, and the prizes are awarded accordingly.

take off just a little more weight, their abdomens will be flat. Some of us find that no matter how thin and muscular we become, our abdomens are still rounded. This is because our beautiful, graceful roundness is not simply caused by fat, it is caused by the underlying structure of our bodies.

I once saw a movie in which a woman entered a beauty contest with the intention of denouncing its sexist and destructive nature. We watch her go through the dehumanizing process of learning to walk like everyone else, learning to smile in the "correct" way, and learning what kinds of attitudes and feelings the judges like. Meanwhile, her feminist supporters keep in touch and get psyched for the planned denunciation. (As I watched it, I was getting pretty psyched myself.) Some time before the contest she practices her intended speech: a glorious critique of the event. She compares the contestants' preparation and showing to the way cattle are bred, herded, judged, and graded.

She wins the contest, but she doesn't give her speech. She has become just like the other contestants. Her acceptance speech is pitiful: without evident intelligence, and certainly without feminist sympathies. This film makes a painful statement regarding the damaging power and influence of objectification, but many viewers wouldn't notice it. The woman is shown making friends with other contestants and enjoying the excitement of the competition. She gets to know the contestants in a genuine, human way. Thus, the true nature of beauty contests is glossed over. Most viewers probably plug in to the traditional excitement of the event and applaud the taming and "success" of this woman.

I wanted to scream my lungs out with the betrayed feminists in the film. Our heroine starts out as an intelligent, independent, and strong individual who knows beauty contests to be degrading and harmful. She has

something important to say: beauty contests dehumanize women. They are a pure form of the objectification that surrounds us every day. But our heroine is not allowed to get her message across because she is brainwashed into celebrating her physical beauty as the measure of her worth.

Pornography is another common form of human objectification. Here again, we are encouraged to look at people as beautiful objects. Much pornography portrays women as defenseless objects to be used and abused for the pleasure of another person or group of people (almost always men). What lies within those beautiful bodies is irrelevant. People are dehumanized, and sexual slavery and abuse is celebrated.

It is obvious that degrading stereotypes of Jews and blacks encourage anti-Semitism and racism. For instance, when blacks are portrayed as shuffling, weak, and stupid characters in the media, racist discrimination is condoned and even encouraged. Whites continue to treat blacks oppressively, and simultaneously blacks internalize inaccurate and destructive self-images. The objectification of women works the same way. Men are taught to treat women as objects, and simultaneously women are taught to think of themselves as objects.

Beauty contests, body-building contests, and pornography are among the purest forms of human objectification. The most insidious offenders, however, are less obvious and most widespread. For example, people are constantly used as sexual objects to sell products in advertising. Bodies or body parts are draped over kitchen appliances and cars like pretty decorations. Beautiful women in revealing clothing tell us about products with seductive voices and expressions. This kind of objectification is so common and "normal" that we hardly notice it.

The cosmetic industry is another insidious influence. It tells us that "beauty" is something every woman can and should buy. It tries to convince us that physical beauty is all-important and that we need an endless array of paints and lotions in order to be beautiful. The commercials instruct us to make ourselves over to cultural images of beauty: "Color your cheeks! Thicken and lengthen your lashes! Cover your blemishes! Brighten your lips!" One would think that we were pieces of furniture in need of refinishing.

Television shows and movies are another showcase for human objectification. The James Bond movies are classic examples of films that objectify masses of women, one after another. Why else do we watch these films except to idolize James Bond, and look at all the beautiful women who parade by, possibly sleep with Bond, and usually do little else? We can choose to avoid such movies; however, most movies have the same type of objectification in smaller doses.

If we are determined to decrease our daily dose of objectification, we can do so. We can avoid beauty contests and body-building contests, for instance, and keep pornography out of our homes. At the same time, however, we must recognize that it is impossible to avoid exposure to objectification unless we avoid contact with virtually everything, including people. Furthermore, avoiding it doesn't change the societal values and practices that cause its proliferation. The underlying values harm us the most. The objectification itself is just a reflection of dehumanizing and sexist values.

What can we do? How can we undermine these destructive influences? The first step consists of an internal decision. Recognizing the damaging influence of objectification can go a long way toward disarming it. For instance, suppose that you are watching television, and across the screen appears an extremely thin, scantily dressed woman. The camera slowly scans her body from her toes to her face, and when it reaches her face, she looks at you as though she's about to take your clothes off and says (very slowly and seductively): "You can never be too rich, or too thin."

Most viewers think: "My god, is she gorgeous! What is she selling?" (And then the answer appears: an airline, a bracelet, or a new television show.) Some viewers will then fantasize about this woman; others will measure themselves against this woman and end up feeling fat and ugly (and, the advertiser hopes, in need of their product). However, any viewer who is aware of the damaging effects of this kind of objectification has a very different reaction: outrage.

Ideally, this commercial can have the opposite of its usual effect. Instead of thinking "I can never be 'too thin,' and I'm certainly not thin enough," a woman may think: "How can anyone put that on TV? Here we are in a culture full of anorexics, bulimics, and chronic dieters who are torturing themselves in the pursuit of these ridiculous aesthetic 'ideals,' and you're telling us that we can never be too thin. What company produced that? I'll never buy their products! I'm going to send them a letter they'll never forget!" Needless to say, someone who has this kind of reaction is not going to be harmed by passive absorption of the damaging messages. Furthermore, if masses of people react this way, advertisers will stop making these harmful commercials. After all, they want to lure, not alienate, potential buyers.

"But those are *just* commercials!" people often point out. "What real harm do they do?" Those commercials actually affect people's behavior. If they didn't, the advertisers wouldn't produce them. The advertisers' goal is to sell products, and they try to lure us to their products with "sexy" bodies. However, I have known many women who rather than (or in addition to) buying products, went on weight-loss diets because they wanted to be as thin as a model or actress whom they saw on television. An especially dramatic example of television's impact involved a recovering anorexic woman. She had regained half of her weight. Then she saw a celebrity on a talk show saying that she always stayed at ninety-five pounds. That week the anorexic woman began to lose all the weight she had gained.

The clothing and fashion industry is another source of destructive messages about women's bodies. First, they all but ignore the needs of fat women. Many Americans require large sizes, but few stores offer a wide selection of large clothing. This increases the pressure to be thin. No one wants to be forced to make clothes, or to pay huge sums to a tailor, or to be stuck with a drab wardrobe. The clothing industry seems to say: "Look, you want to buy clothes? You want a selection? Then lose enough weight to be able to fit into a smaller size." Thus, fat people are denied the right to dress according to personal preference.

Second, women's clothing is ornamentally, rather than instrumentally, designed. Women's comfort and ability to move is not a major concern. High heels, for instance, are not designed or worn for their utility, but rather for their appearance. Girdles and skintight pants are further examples of clothing that is uncomfortable but is nonetheless worn to produce a desired "look." In high heels, girdles, and skintight pants, we cannot run, dance, or even walk freely.

Today and throughout history, women's clothing has had an ornamental rather than instrumental purpose. (In fact, if it has any instrumental purpose, it is to make women physically weaker, less capable, and thereby more dependent and vulnerable.) Consequently, if stylish clothing causes pain or restricted movement, women are supposed to grin and bear it. This is exactly what most women have done in the past and continue to do today. We accept not only society's aesthetic ideals, but *society's judgment that a woman's comfort and ability to function are secondary to her appearance.*

One illustration of this attitude can be found in *Flower of Gold*, a novel about a white woman named Flor de Oro, who was raised by American Indians. As an adult she left Indian society and married a wealthy white man named David Foxcroft. After over four hours of "being worked on" by a dressmaker, hairdresser, and young assistant, she was unveiled to her waiting husband. He exclaimed that she was "the most beautiful woman in the world" and therefore he must be "the most fortunate man on earth." (Meaning that a husband's greatest desire is to have a beautiful wife, and a wife's ultimate value lies in her appearance.)

Learning to Love Our Bodies

"Then I please my husband," she said. "I am happy." (Meaning that as long as she looked beautiful and her husband was pleased, then nothing else mattered to her— she was happy.) David then asked,

"How do you feel?"

The smile in her eyes became a gleam. "Do you really want to know?"

He nodded and the three other women moved forward in anticipation.

Her carriage would have done justice to a queen, her voice was low and decorous. But she said, "Once my people captured a very brave man and thought the manner of his death should equal his courage. He was sewn into a blanket of wet rawhide and placed in the sun. Rawhide is very strong and shrinks much when it dries. He made no cry even as his face turned black and his tongue was forced out of his mouth from the pressure."

She paused and extended a graceful finger of each hand toward her pinched in waist. "I feel just like he did before he died."[7]

David was able to laugh despite the other women's horror and outrage. However, he did not encourage Flor de Oro to wear more comfortable clothing because he nonetheless believed that her appearance was more important than her comfort.

The style of dress depicted in this story is no longer popular: we no longer wear corsets tied so tightly that they crack ribs and damage lungs. However, the same underlying attitude—that a woman's comfort is far less important than her appearance—has not changed. A restrictive diet can be at least as uncomfortable and physically harmful as corsets, and many modern fashions are as painful.

I once asked a friend if I could borrow a pair of her dress shoes. We took the same size, but I decided not to wear any of her shoes because the combination of high heels and narrow toes was very painful. The last pair I tried on were beautiful leather boots. I stood for about three seconds and then sat down for fear of physical damage.

"Aren't they beautiful?" she asked. "They're my favorites. I absolutely love them."

"Yes, they're very attractive," I agreed, "but don't they hurt your feet?"

"Yes," she responded, "but not as much as they used to. The first time I wore them, my feet hurt so much that I cried. I couldn't stop crying until I went home and took them off. But they're not as bad now."

Some women say that their restrictive clothing and high-heeled shoes are not uncomfortable. Many women become accustomed to the discomfort, or build certain muscles (or develop an "adaptive" curve to their spines) and thereby decrease the pain. But the pressure to expect and accept suffering teaches us deeply harmful lessons and priorities. Furthermore, physical damage is usually occurring even though we've become accustomed to the harmful clothing or shoes. High heels strain and damage the spine. They also make it very hard to run (which can be dangerous in certain situations), and increase the probability of ankle sprains.

If you wear uncomfortable clothing, you implicitly accept an ornamental body view, which in turn supports your preoccupation with diet and weight. Furthermore, physical discomfort alienates you from your body, which further supports your preoccupation.

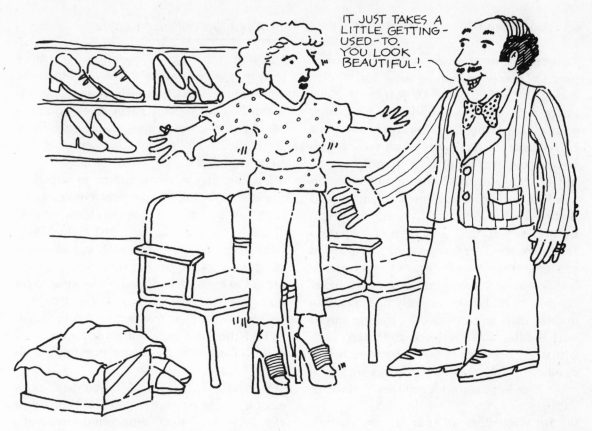

How can you be satisfied and at peace with your body if you are forever feeling physically uncomfortable? Is it strange that when you wear tight clothing you tend to feel "too fat"? In a sense you are, at that moment, too fat: too fat for the clothes you're wearing. But who or what is more important: the clothing or the person who wears it? If the clothing is more important and you exist for the clothing, then you are too fat; but if you are more important and clothing exists to serve you, then *the clothing is too small*.

If you wear tight clothing, then it is perfectly natural and logical that you are "dying to be thinner." Your desire to be thinner not only reflects your pull to conform to aes-

thetic "ideals," it reflects your need for physical comfort. It is virtually impossible to be at peace with your body and wear excessively tight clothing at the same time.

"But I don't want to be at peace with my body!" some of you are thinking. "I don't want to accept my body as it is!" Innumerable sufferers have told me that they cannot allow themselves the comfort of properly sized clothing because they would stop trying to lose (and probably would gain) weight. Thus they reason that their physical discomfort, and the threat of not being able to fit into any of their clothes, pressures them to lose weight. They fear that without this pressure, they will "lose control," give

Learning to Love Our Bodies

up, and continually gain weight until they die.

In order to overcome diet/weight conflict (and the compulsive overeating and undereating that accompany it), you must make peace with your body and stop pressuring yourself to be thin. Dressing comfortably is a prerequisite. In fact, even when your goal is weight loss, uncomfortable clothing undermines your efforts. Constant physical discomfort leads to body preoccupation, and body preoccupation usually leads to weight preoccupation, and weight preoccupation leads to food preoccupation, and food preoccupation leads to desires to eat (regardless of physical need). Furthermore, the discomfort caused by excessively tight clothing and the discomfort caused by hunger can be very similar and therefore confused. Last, physical discomfort leads to feelings of neediness, and one of the ways in which most people nurture themselves is through eating.

"But what does all that matter," people often ask, "if wearing tight clothing motivates me to control my weight?" It's true that given strong enough motivation, people can do just about anything, including kill themselves. But motivating people, including oneself, is not a simple task. *Pressure* often leads to a rebellious reaction: we move in the opposite direction of the pressure in a struggle for freedom and self-determination. Most important, if you are preoccupied with diet and weight, then you have got to take a hard look at *what* you are trying to motivate yourself to do. If you really want to overcome your preoccupation, you will have to stop pressuring yourself to do anything that supports it.

People Objectifying People

The objectification of people is incredibly widespread, not only in the media, but in the way people treat themselves and one another. People objectify themselves, and people objectify other people, all the time. Consequently, the following scene will probably sound familiar.

I was sitting in my living room with two friends, Bob and Janice,[8] watching "Love Boat." A few minutes into the show, we saw "Julie" and some love-at-first-sight lovers talking on the deck. Just as I was about to suggest a game of Backgammon, Janice turned to me and said: "Julie's looking so fat nowadays. She's gained a lot of weight."

"She used to be so attractive," Bob added. "Then they cut her hair and it's been all downhill from there. She's not aging well either."

"Aging?" I thought. "The woman looks about twenty-three. And fat? She's a slender—but not emaciated—woman. Which is to say, of course, that she's 'fat' for an actress."

"Yes, she's looking awful now," Janice agreed.

Next we watched "Fantasy Island." As the fantasizers were getting ready to board the plane and head for home, one of the older actresses entered the picture.

"Do you remember how she used to look?" Janice asked.

"No," I answered. "I don't even know who she is."

"That's (so-and-so)," she informed me (a name I didn't recognize). "She used to be beautiful, but she really let herself go. I can't believe how fat and dumpy she's become."

I must admit that I reacted to these comments with aggravated silence. In retrospect, I wish I had initiated a discussion regarding why, out of all the things they could have criticized or discussed, they chose these two women's appearance. Not the acting, not the script, not the usual ridiculous plots, not something totally unrelated to the tube. Instead, my friends objectified actresses in the usual ways: she's too fat, she's getting old, she's not as attractive as she used to be.

How often do we hear and make this type of comment? They're so common that most people don't notice how much we talk about people's appearance, often without saying anything else about them. Just because we don't notice, however, doesn't mean that this constant drone of objectification doesn't affect the way we think and feel about others and ourselves. When we talk solely about a person's appearance, we indicate that it has primary significance and value— it is the only thing worth commenting on. We imply that appearance is the most important thing to us, and is the basis of our evaluation and thoughts about that person.

Think about the following interchange, which passes between people over and over with small variations.

"Guess who I saw yesterday? . . . Miss Muffet."

"Really? I haven't seen her in years, how's she doing?"

"Pretty well. She looks wonderful: must have lost at least twenty pounds." (They turn to a new topic, this one apparently exhausted.)

When we objectify people, we separate their appearance from their other characteristics. Noticing appearance, in itself, is not problematic. The problem is that we often focus *exclusively* on appearance and categorize a large range of body types as "unattractive." Ideally, appearance would be important, but in a very different way. We would appreciate people's actions, words, ideas, and feelings, and regard their appearance in that light. Appearance is important, but only as part of an inseparable whole.

Have you ever met someone whom you initially found unattractive but later found very attractive? Have you ever met someone whom you initially found very attractive but later found very unattractive? Most of us have had these experiences because people's personalities affect how we "see" them. Anyone we see with love, we see as beautiful.

Appearance is heavily emphasized partly because we see people first and learn about them later. We naturally want to know what to expect from the people we meet, so we try to draw conclusions from the most readily available information. One of the many things I love about George Lucas's *Star Wars* series is the Jedi teaching that appearance often deceives and blinds us. I never tire of hearing Yoda (a great "Jedi Master") say, "Judge me by my size do you? And well you should *not!*"[9] We, who have been taught to assume so much on the basis of body size, would do well to remember that lesson.

THE MEANINGS WE GIVE TO THIN AND FAT

Most of us have a certain image of "the slender, beautiful woman" engraved in our minds: she is lively, popular, successful, sociable, happy, has the man of her dreams, and is in control of herself and her life. This image has little if anything in common with reality, but we carry it around inside us anyway. Should it begin to fade, plenty of advertisements, movies, and people promptly bring it back into focus. For example, most of the advertisements for reducing programs claim that by losing weight, "you too" can attain a new outlook, a better social life, a perfect man, greater enjoyment, fulfillment, and, in effect, a new and better "you."

Being fat has also come to mean a lot more than having a fat body. Many consider fatness a sign of laziness, gluttony, lack of self-control, lack of self-esteem, gullibility, psychological conflict, and even stupidity.[10] Fat people suffer from discrimination similar to other forms of minority discrimination. Fat children are teased and rejected by their peers;[11] fat people are less often accepted by colleges than are their equally qualified but thinner peers;[12] and fat people often suffer from job discrimination.[13] Most of us either consciously or unconsciously accept and apply a negative stereotype to fat people. Thus, our society is not only sexist and racist, but "fattist" as well.

Some of the most wonderful, warm, and well-meaning people are fattist without realizing it. But fattism is no more justifiable than racism or sexism. It is irrational prejudice based on physical characteristics. Nonetheless, fattism is extremely widespread and a *socially acceptable* form of prejudice. One can walk into a room and say, "Look at all those disgusting fat slobs." Equivalent racist comments are considered much less acceptable; hopefully fattist comments will soon be socially unacceptable as well.

The meanings and characteristics most of us attach to slenderness and fatness increase our desire to avoid being fat at any cost. We want to become like the slender images that are so consistently celebrated, and we are terrified of becoming like the fat images that are so consistently degraded.

Parents often encourage this fear. I have worked with many women who have been pressured to lose weight by their parents even though they were never overweight by medical standards. The pressure is sometimes incredibly intense. One woman I know was constantly goaded by her mother (who, incidentally, was a clinical psychologist). When she finally lost her "extra" fifteen pounds, she was rewarded with a new wardrobe and a party to celebrate her new figure. Furthermore, every time this woman spoke to her mother on the phone, she was asked to report on her weight!

Another woman's father often said she could "accomplish anything" she wanted if she could just lose weight. She was about twenty pounds heavier than "model thin." How her father managed to make the "logical" leap, skip, and jump from losing weight to omnipotence, she didn't know. Nonetheless, his statement, repeated over the years, helped to convince this young woman that being "fat" was her most debilitating obstacle.

One of the many reasons why this father's statement was so harmful is that it encouraged his daughter to have "illusions of slender grandeur." Unfortunately, his statement is simply another version of what most weight-loss programs claim to provide. "If only I were thin I would be perfect and my life would be wonderful." This sounds like the statement of a raving lunatic when you consider it rationally, but many people have been brainwashed into believing it.

How many of us question the value of a weight-loss diet for "self-improvement"? Who among us has never gone on a diet in response to negative feelings about ourselves and/or our lives? Whenever I ask an audience to raise their hands if they've ever gone on a weight-loss diet to "improve themselves," virtually every hand goes right up. Think about the implicit value judgment which underlies that behavior. The assumption is that thin people are *better* than fat people, and therefore anyone who loses weight automatically becomes a better person.

We have our values all screwed around. We could use our energy to love one another more fully, but instead we focus on weight loss. We could learn to sing or dance, or be more understanding and patient. The options are endless, but instead we focus on weight loss. Imagine how different things would be if all the psychological time and energy that now goes into obsessing about our bodies were focused on loving ourselves and one another.

But we don't seem to believe that one can become "better" or happier by practicing the art of loving fully, being honest with ourselves and others, and building supportive relationships. We believe what the media tell us: that the best road to self-improvement and happiness is an effective weight-loss program.

ANOREXIC THOUGHTS AND ATTITUDES

By now I hope that at least this much is clear: we have got to begin to question and amend the way we think about our bodies, other people's bodies, and what we value in people. So many people are being harmed by this craziness. As long as we think and act like everyone else, we are part of the problem. When we begin to think and behave differently—when we refuse to be fattist and are fat-supportive; when we refuse to objectify people and, instead, appreciate people in humanistic ways; when we oppose, instead of conform to, harmful prescriptive norms—then we will help not only ourselves, but all of the people around us.

How destructive are our priorities and our thinking? Very destructive. Most people who are preoccupied with diet and weight have what I would call "anorexic" tendencies. *Not* that they are in danger of becoming anorexic—most aren't. But they have harmful "anorexic thoughts," and a bizarre "respect" for anorexic behavior. These attitudes encourage self-destructiveness, and make it harder for anorexics to give up their self-starvation to choose life over a living (or actual) death.

One afternoon I was working as a security guard (a great temporary job for a writer), when some executives were getting ready to leave the building. The head honcho, a very nice woman, asked how my book was coming along. We'd already talked about my work, so she knew what it was about.

As she was leaving, she said, "You know, I wish I could get anorexia."

Learning to Love Our Bodies

She wasn't the first to say this to me (far from it), so I used a well-worn response: "You don't really, do you?" But she assured me in no uncertain terms that she *did* want to be anorexic. She wanted to be anorexic so that she wouldn't be overweight.

This woman was not model slim; however, she wasn't particularly overweight either. I'd guess that she had the usual desire to lose about twenty pounds. Obviously, she didn't know what it would be like to be anorexic. If she had, she wouldn't have wanted the illness. Nonetheless, it's amazing that this intelligent, highly successful executive would rather be dangerously underweight—totally emaciated—than be twenty pounds heavier than she considered aesthetically ideal.

I have found that this is a common attitude. When I speak for women's groups on diet/weight conflict and eating disorders, I often try a quick experiment:

"On the paper in front of you, write down a weight you would *really* like to maintain—a weight you consider ideal for yourself. Now subtract twelve pounds from that number and circle the new amount. Okay, leave that for now and add twelve pounds to your chosen ideal weight and circle the sum. . . . If you had the choice, right now, of weighing one or the other of these weights you've just circled, which would you choose? . . . How many of you would choose the higher weight?" (Very few people, invariably, raise their hands.)

"How many of you would choose the lower weight?" (70–100 percent of the audience raise their hands.)

"Would you be healthier at the higher or lower weight?" (We eventually establish that the higher weights are healthier.)

"Knowing this, and taking it into consideration, ask yourself the same question: would you rather be at the lighter or the heavier weight?" (Everyone sort of shakes her head and maybe smiles or laughs nervously and admits that she would still prefer to be emaciated rather than twelve pounds "too heavy.")

Female audiences almost always demonstrate two points. First, most young women have "anorexic thoughts" and attitudes. Second, and in a sense more important, the whole diet, exercise, and weight fad in this country is primarily motivated by *aesthetic ideals* and people's strong desire to "look good" rather than by desires for better health or longer life. Everyone is dying to be "beautiful." If they can be healthy at the same time, they love it. If they have to exchange their health for "beauty," they still consider it a bargain.

Think about it.

The combination of fattism, ornamental body views, objectification, and the idealization of slenderness cause a great many women to focus on their appearance as the most important aspect of themselves, and to focus on their degree of slenderness as the most important aspect of their appearance. Even if a woman rejects these societal judgments on an intellectual level, her desire to be very slim does not readily disappear. This is the first seed of diet/weight conflict and eating disorders: a strong desire to be very thin.

You need to let go of this self-destructive desire. Unfortunately, it is the most difficult symptom to give up because the social rewards for being very thin (and punishment for being fat) constantly support excessively slender goals and diet/weight conflict. Thus you may feel as though you are trapped in a no-win situation: if you continue to struggle with your body, you will continue to suffer the resulting physical and psychological pain; if you make peace with your body, you will be less "beautiful" according to prevailing aesthetic ideals.

I cannot deny that our society rewards slenderness—it does. However, the rewards for making peace with your body are far greater:

1. It is relatively easy to live well and be happy while enjoying physical comfort and good health; it is virtually impossible to live well and be happy while struggling against your body's basic physical needs.

2. When we learn to fill our physical needs, we learn to respect and take care of ourselves. We may have to stand up to social pressure to conform, but we can struggle against externally imposed problems and be at peace with ourselves. We cannot struggle against *ourselves* and be at peace.

3. If we direct our energy toward creating an environment that encourages sane, life-supportive values, then we direct our energy toward something constructive. Progress is a likely result. If we channel our energy toward conforming to destructive values, then we support the values that are destroying us. Progress is simply impossible.

4. When considering the pros and cons of pursuing a slender body, beware of assuming that the choice is between (a) *being thin* and physically and psychologically at war with yourself, and (b) being "fatter" and physically at peace. If you are like 99 percent of the people who struggle to control their weight, that is *not* the true choice. Why? Because under choice (a) you will not "be thin" most of the time. Your struggles will result in yo-yoing (and possibly escalating) weight rather than slenderness. Thus, the choice is more likely (a) being heavier than aesthetic ideals most of the time and physically and psychologically at war with yourself, and (b) being heavier than aesthetic ideals all of the time, and physically (and eventually psychologically) at peace.

Once upon a time (too short a time ago), I decided to allow my body to be whatever size it was meant to be. I was maintaining my weight below 100 pounds when I made that decision, though I had once weighed about 130 pounds. I didn't know how fat I would become, but I knew that I would eventually weigh over 110 pounds. Even 110 seemed unbearably high; nonetheless, I let my slenderness go.

As I became heavier, I felt more scared and upset with every pound. And when my periods returned, I cried with despair. Nonetheless, I kept working toward freedom, because I finally wanted it even more than I wanted to be thin.

Deep inside, underneath the destructive lessons and the ways in which we've been hurt, we all want peace of mind and body. Deep down, we all know that this is far more important than being thin. The process toward this state of peace and freedom can be incredibly painful, but the rewards are well worth our trouble.

As you work through and let go of your self-destructive desires and values, you too may feel scared and upset. Don't push yourself too hard. Use the suggestions (below) that you are ready to use and let the others wait. You have plenty of time, and later chapters will help you build strong self-esteem that is not dependent on your weight. Don't try to give up your old destructive goals and behavior until you are able to *replace them* with new constructive goals and behavior. Don't follow any suggestion in this book until you feel ready— you always have the option of coming back to it later.

DEVELOPING POSITIVE BODY AWARENESS

You probably think about how thin or fat you are every day. You may weigh yourself every day (or even many times a day) in order to monitor even the slightest weight fluctuation. Or you may not know your weight in terms of a number on a scale, yet "feel" and look for weight fluctuations. Thus, in one way or another, you are probably acutely aware of how fat or thin you are. The primary reason for this kind of body awareness is a strong desire to be conventionally attractive or "sexy." In other words, you view your body in an ornamental way, and you idealize slenderness.

In order to gain freedom from this preoccupation, you need to change your body view. For instance, you need to be more concerned with how you feel than with how fat or thin you look. If you are one of the many sufferers who are addicted to using a scale, the first step is to *stop weighing yourself.* Why? Because whenever you get on that scale, you are going to judge your body, and probably yourself, on the basis of weight. You will thus support your ornamental body view and your preoccupation with weight, all of which are destructive. You need to learn that you are far more than a number on a scale.

Many people who are preoccupied with diet and weight constantly look at their bodies (I call them "lookers"), while others constantly avoid seeing their bodies ("avoiders"). If you are in the habit of scrutinizing your body at every opportunity, then stop doing it. For when you look at yourself at home in your mirror, and in store windows, car windows, public restroom mirrors, and every other reflective object that comes your way, you are probably looking to see how fat you appear. You are objectifying yourself.

Your body is much more than a beautiful object. So when you're tempted to look in a store window to see how you look, look at the people, plants, buildings, and trees around you instead. Think about how you feel instead of how you look. Do you feel like you're ready to "leap over tall buildings in a single bound," or do you feel as though you can barely move (or somewhere in between)? Are you ready to take a step toward one of your goals, or are you feeling unable to deal with challenges just now? Breaking the habit of constantly looking at yourself will take time and effort. You can start undoing your appearance obsession by putting any especially tempting mirrors you have in your house (a large mirror in your bedroom, for example) into storage.

If, on the other hand, you avoid looking at your body—probably because you are afraid of what you might see—then it is time to take off all your clothes and stand in front of a full-length mirror. First concentrate on what you like about your body. Your body cannot be all "bad" even from your prejudiced viewpoint. Feel the texture of your skin. How do you like it? Next look at the parts of your body you most dislike. Why do you dislike them? Are your reasons ornamental or instrumental? *Is the "badness" or "unattractiveness" real, or just a figment of your aesthetically thin mind?*

None of us will ever stop wanting to be attractive. That's not the problem. The problem is that we consider slender bodies, and only slender bodies, attractive. Soft, full, curving figures are in reality as beautiful as any other kind. While you work toward a more instrumental body view, work also for an expanded aesthetic appreciation of the human body. Notice beauty in all different bodies, including your own. Let your eyes continue to be caught by large, fatter-than-average people; but instead of measuring yourself against their bodies, and instead of thanking God that you are not that large or cursing yourself because you are, look for and admire their special beauty. If given the opportunity, meet them—find out who you're looking at—because who they are is an inseparable part of their beauty.

After you do the mirror exercise, switch over to thinking about your body in an *instrumental* way. Chances are that your body is serving most of your needs quite admirably. Appreciate how well it functions for you, and how much pleasure it can give you.

This brings us to a very important topic: sexuality. In order to make peace with your body, you must learn about your sexuality and become a fully responsive, sensual, orgasmic person. If you have never masturbated to orgasm, learn to do so, and enjoy it often. (Lonnie Barbach's *For Yourself* is a helpful guide for preorgasmic women. See Resources, p. 240.) You deserve complete sexual pleasure, and that pleasure will help you appreciate your body as a dear friend. Your body (and the way you have treated it) has caused you physical and mental torment. It's time to be nice to your body. It's time to learn to enjoy your body to the fullest!

If you are a sexually active woman who rarely (if ever) has orgasms, realize here and now that the female body is not designed to be stimulated by purely "vaginal" intercourse. Only a small minority of women reach orgasm from the stimulation provided by "traditional" coitus. This is *not* because women are "frigid." It is because we require clitoral stimulation to experience full pleasure, and the clitoris is not in the vagina. If you are not enjoying orgasms on a regular basis (and it doesn't matter if you have no partners, one, or many, or whether you're homosexual, bisexual, or heterosexual), figure out what you need to fully enjoy your sexuality. Find an instructive self-help book, expand your sexual fantasizing, join a sexuality workshop, and practice! If you have a lover, get him/her involved. She/he needs

Learning to Love Our Bodies

to understand your body and know your needs and desires, too.

If you are one of the many women who were sexually abused at a young age, issues surrounding your sexuality will be difficult and painful. In addition, you may find that your eating problems are strongly connected with your traumatic experiences as a child or adolescent. For instance, a woman who has been sexually abused sometimes tries to protect herself from sexual advances by overeating and gaining weight or by starving herself and thereby refusing to develop a mature woman's body. Other times, an eating disorder can be used to dull unbearable feelings or to keep one's focus on food, eating, and weight, and thereby avoid the more painful issues.

If you have been sexually abused, I strongly recommend that you read *The Courage to Heal: A Guide for Women Survivors of Child Sexual Abuse* (see Resources, p. 242). Regardless of whether or not these experiences relate to your struggle with food and weight, you will find this an extremely supportive and helpful book.

Last but not least, every female reader should know that if you suffer from menstrual cramps, you are probably suffering unnecessarily. See (or call) your gynecologist right away and ask for relief. She may prescribe Motrin, or suggest that you use Advil, Nuprin, or some other drug that relieves menstrual cramps. Or see a chiropractor, acupuncturist, or masseuse for alternative remedies. There is nothing quite like monthly pain to alienate you from your own body and womanhood! Don't suffer from it if you don't have to.

As we discussed earlier, clothing can have a tremendous effect on the way you feel about your body. To review and summarize, uncomfortable clothing or shoes will reinforce your preoccupation with diet and weight—not only because you are conforming to (and thereby supporting) a harmful value, but because uncomfortable clothing alienates you from your body.

The more physical discomfort you experience, the more you and your body will seem to be at odds. How can you like your body if you are usually uncomfortable? If you wear tight and restrictive clothing, you will feel too fat. If you cannot walk very far or dance for very long before your feet, ankles, and possibly back hurt from the strain of moving in high-heeled shoes, then you are likely to feel hampered by your body. If you dress as though being conventionally attractive is more important than anything else, then you will feel dehumanized.

Try to increase your physical pleasure and decrease your physical discomfort as much as possible. Also, experiment with doing the opposite of some of the things you do now. For instance, if you are a "looker," stop looking at yourself so much. If you are an "avoider," confront and admire yourself in a mirror. If you tend to wear tight clothing and high heels, try wearing something different. If you always hide your body in very loose clothing, try wearing something closer fitting but still comfortable. If you never "dress up," then try dressing up. By changing these seemingly minor habits, you will force yourself to question what you've been doing and take the risk of confirming or disproving your assumptions and fears. Thinking about and deciding to make a change is nearly always more difficult and painful than the change itself. So go ahead—make a small change in your life!

REGULAR EXERCISE

I have hesitated to emphasize the helpfulness of exercise because people who are preoccupied with diet and weight often use it in a destructive way. Most of us have tried to use exercise to lose weight. Many people —mostly men—feel that they have to be athletic and muscular in order to be "attractive." The common presumptions that we are inadequate unless we exercise regularly, or unless we are muscular, or unless we are coordinated, or unless we are thin, are *all* oppressive. As I discuss the ways in which exercise can help you let go of your preoccupation, remember that I am *not* saying that everyone should exercise regularly, or that everyone should be athletic. Our physical activity level is not a moral issue. Plenty of wonderful people enjoy sedentary lives. Their choice of life-style is perfectly legitimate.

One of the most effective ways to let go of your exclusively ornamental body view is to develop a more instrumental body view. Physical exercise can be used to do this. Through exercise you can begin to appreciate your ability to move and "play" as well as your physical beauty. As you discover the joy of movement (and perhaps sport), you will also come to *feel better*—and the better you feel (physically), the more at peace you will feel with your physical self.

Through exercise you can become less hampered by physical limitations and thereby feel more at home in your body. Just going up a few flights of stairs, moving a full trash can, or dashing for a departing bus can be unpleasant if you do not have the strength to do it with ease. These kinds of movement are basic to most people's lives. We don't need to be very strong to feel able-bodied in the modern world, but because we are required to exercise very little, it is easy to become uncomfortably weak and thereby alienated from our bodies.

Most of you have used exercise as part of a reducing regimen; consequently, you have focused on calories burned and pounds lost. An exercise program designed to undermine diet/weight conflict must have completely different goals, such as:

1. to have fun

2. to feel better physically and mentally

3. to promote a less ornamental and more instrumental body view

4. to develop unconditional body acceptance and appreciation

5. to improve health

What happened to number 6: to lower set-point weight? That goal, in itself, can be very harmful. Regular exercise often leads to a lower weight, but weight loss does not determine the value of an exercise program. An exercise program will help you overcome diet/weight conflict *if* your primary goals are to feel better, to change your body view, and to gain strength. Fitness and leanness are *not* the same thing!

In order to use exercise in a helpful way, I

suggest that you try to exercise regularly: set a goal of three workouts per week. Try to spread your exercise out rather than exercising on consecutive days. That way your body will have time to recover after each workout, and you will be less likely to hurt yourself. You don't have to follow a rigid program: exercise more often than planned whenever you want to, and don't condemn yourself if you don't manage to get in all three workouts. However, remember that regularity makes an exercise program easier to maintain. You can decide when to exercise in advance, put that time aside in your schedule, and avoid constantly asking yourself, "Shall I exercise today or not?"

If you stop exercising for a long period of time, there is no need to feel guilty. It happens to everyone, and feeling bad about it is unproductive. Remember that you are still the same person you were while exercising —lack of exercise has made you less fit, *not* less worthy. Just as eating poorly does not make you a "bad" person, failing to exercise does not make you a "bad" person. Ideally, you should handle it in the same way most people who love to be active handle it: mildly regret that you don't feel as good because of inactivity; mildly regret that you haven't been enjoying the fun and mental relaxation you had been enjoying; and go back to it as soon as you can.

If you are out of shape, start out slowly: don't push yourself too hard, and ask a doctor if she foresees any special problems. Everyone has a different idea about what constitutes "too much." Muscle builders, for instance, use the guideline "No pain, no gain." Your guideline should be very different from that. If your goals are enjoyment, greater appreciation for your body, and improved fitness and health, there is no need for discomfort.

"Discomfort" in this context does not refer to the minor feelings of fatigue and strain that inevitably come and go as you exercise. However, if you feel terrible when you run (for instance), try running more slowly or walking. Always look for the most comfortable pace for everything you do. Make enjoyment your first priority. You can most readily attain the goals listed above through painless, enjoyable exercise.

Last spring a friend of mine from college, Dan, was talking about runners who wear small tape players or radios. He disapproved because he felt that music would make it "too easy and pleasant" and thereby destroy the psychological benefits. "If you don't think about your breathing and pace and pain, then what's the point?" In the ensuing argument, Dan said that if he wasn't in pain, then he wasn't pushing himself hard enough. But at the time of this conversation, Dan had driven himself away from exercise, for he was sedentary. Do not fall into the trap of pushing yourself so hard that you push yourself away from the fun of exercise.

What kind of exercise should you do? Any form of exercise that you can and like to do. The ultimate goal is to participate in every form of exercise you enjoy and none of the forms you don't enjoy. Explore as many options as you can. Even if you find only one or two forms that you really love, the time and effort you spend searching will be well spent. Recreational exercise will enrich your life in many ways. Not only will it be fun and help you stay fit, it will help you relax. If you enjoy recreational exercise on a regular basis, you cannot help but enjoy improved physical and mental well-being as side effects.

Here are a few forms of exercise you might like to try:

Walking

Walking is probably the most natural form of exercise because that is how we are designed to move around. Use it as a form of transportation (whenever you can make the time), and it will be especially satisfying. Walking is a good beginning if you haven't been exercising much, but be sure to wear shoes with enough support.

Do you ever cruise around parking lots in search of a space near the door? Most of us do it even though it's a remarkably silly habit. Park far away where there are plenty of spaces. You will not only save time and gas, but you will probably feel better when you reach the door.

The natural extension of walking is hiking. Day hikes are a wonderful way to spend time with a friend: pack a lunch and go for it. With a close friend it hardly matters where you walk because the enjoyment will come from being together and from moving around. Of course, it's nice to go somewhere pretty. Hiking in the mountains for a weekend or longer requires equipment and know-how. If possible, find a friend to take you on your first trip. Otherwise, many books are available for learning about and planning a backpacking trip. Backpacking is very satisfying if you are in good physical condition; however, if you're out of shape, be very careful not to push yourself, or it will become a form of torture. Hike only as much as feels comfortable.

Running

Needless to say, running is very popular these days. It is inexpensive, does not require a partner or team, can be done any day (as long as you don't mind inclement weather), and has far-reaching benefits.

Running is great for your lungs and cardiovascular system but *very bad for your joints*. Most people run on pavement, which leads to harmful pounding. Be sure to wear good running sneakers to decrease the impact, and, when possible, run on grass or dirt. If you choose to run on a regular basis, keep in mind that you can hurt yourself despite precautions. If you feel pain in any of your joints (knees or ankles, for example), stop running immediately.

Many people find running boring. You might like to carry a small radio or tape player with lightweight headphones. Or try to develop an appreciation for the meditative quality of running. If you still don't enjoy running, don't run—find some other form of exercise to enjoy.

Dancing

Dancing is all about the joy of movement. With or without instruction, most people find that moving their bodies to music feels great. Dance does not require a large investment in equipment or fees, so virtually anyone can do it. The biggest block to enjoying dance is embarrassment and lack of confidence. There are lots of ways to let go of those feelings. Watch a random group of people dance at a social event. Notice the people who are obviously enjoying themselves. They look wonderful whether or not they have any dance training (or sense of rhythm, for that matter). They're having a great time! If you are still afraid to dance in public, dance at home to a radio or stereo until you feel more confident.

Try many forms of dance. For instance, look for square dances and folk dances in a local paper. Many are designed for beginners (particularly during the early part of the dance), so that teaching is included. If you would feel more comfortable in a class (and have the time and money), try that. In the long run, aim for a form of dance you can do on a regular basis without having to depend on classes. You'll find it cheaper and more likely to become a lasting form of entertainment and exercise.

Many exercise spas offer "aerobic dance" classes and other forms of structured exercise classes. These can be enjoyable and convenient; but be careful *not* to use an establishment designed to help people lose weight. (Unfortunately, most spas and clubs fall into this category because weight reducers provide an enormous market.) If you join a spa that stresses weight reduction and appearance, your exercise program will support your preoccupation. If you have the strength to participate while insisting that you have no interest in losing weight—go ahead. You will rock everyone's boat in a fantastic way! However, *beware:* if the attitudes of all the figure-obsessed staff and members begin to affect you, get out immediately. Find a supportive place to exercise and have fun.

Swimming

Swimming is an excellent form of exercise. It utilizes virtually every muscle in your body without straining joints. At certain spots you can swim for free. Many hotels allow the public to use their pools for a small fee. Many towns offer inexpensive indoor swimming. If swimming is difficult for you, a little instruction can go a long way toward increasing your stamina and enjoyment.

Cycling

Riding a bike is not only a wonderful form of exercise, it can be a very useful form of transportation. Many people who do not have cars get along by walking, taking public transportation, and riding a bike. In cities one can often go from one place to another as quickly on a bike as in a car, and bikes are much easier to park. Of course, even a used bike requires an investment; but with proper care a bike lasts a long time, and the cost of maintenance is low.

Do not ride long distances without working up to it slowly or you will promptly turn yourself off to long-distance riding. Long-distance riding is a great way to spend a vacation. You can stay and (usually) cook your breakfasts and dinners at very inexpensive hostels.[14]

These five suggestions only scratch the surface of an infinite number of possibilities. I've left out many popular individual and partner activities, and I've left out team sports altogether. Make up your own list.

You need not exercise for the same amount of time every workout. Sometimes you will be able to exercise all day. Other days it may be difficult to squeeze in half an hour. Some days you will feel especially energetic and want to exercise long and hard. Other days you will feel lazy. You need not push yourself when you're feeling lazy, but try not to skip a planned workout altogether. A little exercise can make you feel more energetic.

Finding time to exercise regularly is not easy if you work forty or more hours per week. You'll need motivation, determination, and positive reinforcement. Having fun and feeling good will provide some incentive, but additional reinforcement is helpful. Sharing your exercise program with someone else, particularly if she has similar goals, adds vital support. Do not share your exercise program, however, with someone who is trying to lose weight.

You can also provide positive reinforcement for yourself by keeping an exercise journal. Journal entries can entail anything from a three-work report of what you did to pages of comments on how much you enjoyed yourself, how you feel, how much

your stamina has increased, and what goals you would like to reach and why. Include anything that seems important to you. You can use longer journal entries as an outlet for bad feelings as well as a place to revel in good feelings. The journal can also help you *focus on instrumental concerns.* Avoid focusing on your appearance or weight. Do not let negative goals that will support diet/weight conflict take the place of your original goals.

Exercise will help you appreciate and enjoy your body *if* you approach it with those goals in mind. Even as you try to use it in this way, people will assume and encourage you to believe that the primary purpose of exercise is weight loss and control. Consequently, you must be careful to use it as a way to have fun, to feel better, and to develop a more instrumental body view. An exclusively ornamental body view leads to pain and alienation regardless of how you look. Once your body is a major source of fun and pleasure, you will automatically appreciate it. Your body is your home. Your body is an integral part of yourself. You deserve to appreciate and enjoy your body whether you are fat or thin or somewhere in between.

IMPORTANT GOALS TO KEEP IN MIND

1. See your body as a trusted and treasured home for yourself to enjoy and use fully, rather than as an aesthetic object.

2. Enrich and broaden your aesthetically thin mind: notice beauty in everyone around you.

3. Replace fattism with respect for all people regardless of size.

4. See people as whole human beings, rather than objects with certain physical characteristics.

5. Stop weighing yourself. Get rid of your scale if you have one.

6. Stop using your weight and weight control as a measure of your value; value yourself simply for who you are.

7. Clothe yourself comfortably and pleasingly, knowing that you deserve to be comfortable.

8. Increase your physical pleasure and decrease your physical discomfort as much as possible.

9. Reject the destructive social prescription to be as thin as possible in your every thought, word, and action.

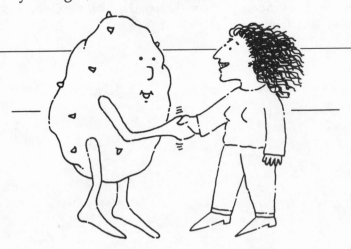

PERSONAL QUESTIONS:
TRANSFORMING YOUR BODY IMAGE

1. What did you think about your body *before* you began to worry about diet and weight? Did you like your body? Why or why not? When did you learn to worry about your diet and weight?

2. How often do you weigh yourself?

3. If you weigh yourself frequently, how do you think it affects you?

- Set a goal to stop weighing yourself by a certain realistic date:

- What steps must you take to reach your goal?

4. Are you a "looker" or an "avoider" (or a combination)? How does frequently looking at yourself, or avoiding the sight of your body, support your diet/weight obsession?

Learning to Love Our Bodies

- Set a specific goal to change your pattern by a certain realistic date:

- What steps must you take to reach your goal?

5. Do you hide yourself in very baggy or unexciting clothing? If so, why? How does this affect your feelings about yourself? When and how would you like to change this pattern?

6. How often, if ever, do you wear clothing or shoes that are uncomfortable (and even physically harmful)? How does this affect you? When can you begin to change this?

7. Do you own clothing that will not fit unless you are under your setpoint weight? If so, how does this affect you? What can you do about it?

8. What changes in the way you dress would help you undermine your preoccupation with diet and weight?

- Set specific goals:

• What steps must you take to reach your goals?

9. How do you judge other people on the basis of their appearance? For instance, do you respect fat people less than thin people? If so, do you consider it fair or just?

10. How do you apply fattism to yourself? Do you believe that you are (or would be) "better" or more capable if thinner? Why or why not?

11. To what extent do you judge yourself solely on the basis of your appearance? Are you harder on yourself than on others? If so, why?

12. Do you behave differently depending on what you weigh? If so, in what ways? When can you begin to act as you like, regardless of what you weigh?

13. How does a bony body versus a fatter body feel to your touch? What is pleasant and what is unpleasant about each one? Now answer from an infant's point of view. Which would an infant find more pleasant?

14. Do you have a primarily ornamental or instrumental body view? List three things you can do in order to develop (or enhance) an instrumental body view.

a.

b.

c.

15.   Make a list of what you like about yourself and your recent accomplishments that have nothing to do with appearance.

WHAT I LIKE ABOUT MYSELF	ACCOMPLISHMENTS

16.   Do you exercise regularly? If not, what gets in your way? Do you enjoy exercising?

17.   Do you feel that a regular exercise program can help you to undermine your preoccupation? Why or why not? (If not, skip to question 21.)

18.   Make a list of every physically demanding activity you can think of. Put a check next to all the activities you enjoy and a T for "try it out" next to all those you have never tried.

	ACTIVITY		ACTIVITY

19.   How can it help you to expand the number of physically demanding activities you do and enjoy? Draw up a plan for accomplishing this goal. For instance, what new activity would you like to try first? When can you try it?

20. If you want to begin a regular exercise program, make a list of your goals and your game plan for achieving them.

- Set specific goals:

- What resources do you have to help you? Are you going to share your exercise program with anyone? Do you want to keep a journal?

- What will your challenges be? What will oppose your efforts?

- What steps must you take to reach your goals?

21. Think of at least three specific things you can do to try to counteract societal influences that support diet/weight preoccupation.

a. I can

b. I can

c. I can

22. How are you feeling about your body right now? Why?

23. How are you feeling about yourself right now? Why?

24. Imagine that you are completely at peace with your body and yourself—that you really love and appreciate the person you are to the fullest. Describe what you think and feel about yourself and your body, in the present tense, as if it were true.

25. Write down at least four things you like about your body. Let yourself feel really good about those things—knowing that your body *is* worthy of unqualified appreciation.

    a.

    b.

    c.

    d.

26. Write down at least four things you like about yourself. Let yourself feel really good about those things—knowing that you are worthy of respect, love, and unqualified appreciation.

    a.

    b.

    c.

    d.

4

LEARNING TO EAT SPONTANEOUSLY

On the way home I drew up my plan. I would stick to my rigid diet for the first week—no exceptions no matter what; then I would eat all weekend at the parties and family get-togethers; and during the final week I would go back to the diet and recoup my losses.

The first week was no problem. Did I want some ice cream, my mother wanted to know? No, I can't have ice cream. Everything was resisted unless it was part of the program. I was so good that I lost another pound.

Then the weekend: endless partying, drinking, and bingeing. I went totally wild: cheesecake, ice cream, muffins, beer, quiche, cookies ... everything I wanted. On Sunday night I indulged in the final binge: Chinese food, popcorn at the movies, and a midnight snack. I was so bad—but I just had to eat. Then, of course, it was all over. As I went to bed I fought my guilt and fear by planning the coming week's deprivation, but I cried myself to sleep.

A VACATION IN THE LIFE OF A CHRONIC DIETER

Once upon a time, women ate when they felt hungry. These days, most of us suspect that we feel hungry when we're not "really hungry"; or that we want to eat when we're not hungry; or that we're always (or never) hungry! We are told that excessive hunger is evidence of unfulfilled emotional or sexual needs, boredom, or depression. Hunger has become our enemy. We try to destroy it through appetite suppressants, deny it through mind control, and trick it through bizarre diets and noncaloric "foods." We are afraid we will lose control and gorge ourselves—become victims of our insatiable and unbearable hunger.

But let's step back a moment. What did hunger mean to us *before* we became consumed with diet and weight? What was our hunger like, and what did we think about eating?

All of us were born without any questions about hunger. I used to swallow (not eat—swallow) breakfast as I watched my school bus cruise down the street. I consumed it because it was served—no decision involved, no big deal. At school I ate a bag lunch—again as a matter of course. When I arrived home, the first order of business was a snack. I would eat toast with butter and cinnamon-sugar until I was tired of it. If that meant one slice, fine. If that meant four slices, fine. I didn't care because it never did me any harm. My siblings began to call me "toast lady," but they never saw anything wrong with my consumption of bread, butter, cinnamon, and sugar—it was just an amusing idiosyncrasy. At dinner I'd eat a small meal and then try to choose the optimal moment to ask to be excused.

As a child, I *didn't think* about eating. I ate as unconsciously as I slept or went to the bathroom. The end of a meal was natural and unconflicted. I never thought, "Do I deserve more?" or "Can I resist eating more?" or "When will I eat again?" I never thought, "Have I been good today?" or "How many calories is this?" My eating occasionally became a conflict between me and my parents (when they forced me to eat liver, for instance), but eating was *never* a conflict between me and myself. I hadn't even conceived of such a thing.

Most of us enjoyed a time when hunger was simply hunger. We could easily tell when we were hungry; we knew that it was normal and natural to feel hungry many times every day; and we knew how to satisfy our hunger. This is what we must relearn: a natural, relaxed, unconflicted, and spontaneous way of eating. Unfortunately, there is no instant way to replace conflicted eating with spontaneous eating. Before that exchange can take place, we must let go of our fear—our fear of hunger and food. We must

first understand our hunger, then befriend it, and *then* stop worrying about it.

Most people assume that if their stomachs are empty, they're likely to be hungry, and if their stomachs are full, they "should" feel sated. These assumptions seem logical, but they reflect a simplistic and inaccurate understanding of hunger. *Hunger is not governed by our stomachs.*

Unfortunately, even physiologists don't fully understand hunger. Certain regions of the brain seem to regulate hunger, and glucose levels in the blood affect hunger; however, *there is no known way to tell whether a given experience of hunger is "real" (physiologically induced) or imaginary.*

We nonetheless assume that these two kinds of hunger exist: real hunger and imaginary hunger. I call the first kind "body hunger" because the hunger is caused by our bodies' need for food. I call all other kinds of hunger "mind hunger."

Any desire to eat in the absence of body hunger is mind hunger (some people call it "appetite"), and everyone experiences it. For instance, suppose you just ate a fairly large meal and feel sated, but just as you're about to leave the table, your favorite dessert arrives. Unless you're already stuffed (and possibly even then), you're likely to want some. Or suppose you are bored or tired—you may relieve the boredom or gain energy by eating. I have yet to meet anyone who has never, for one reason or another, eaten without "really feeling hungry." Everyone experiences and responds to mind hunger. You don't have to be a compulsive overeater to eat when you're not hungry.

Mind hunger also refers to mistaken instances of hunger: you think you're hungry when, in fact, no body hunger exists. We can mistake other sensations, such as feeling tired or cold, for hunger. We can mistake an emotion, such as loneliness or anxiety, for hunger. In theory, any physical sensation or emotion can be a source of mind hunger.

Dr. Hilde Bruch refers to our ability to identify and differentiate body hunger from other states of mind and body as our "hunger awareness." She argues that while body hunger is an automatic response to a need for nourishment, our ability to *identify* body hunger is learned. Some people learn it well, others don't. Those who don't, she says, have faulty hunger awareness.

People with faulty hunger awareness may never feel hungry, or never feel sated, or mistake mind hunger for body hunger, or simply be unable to identify hunger. Dr. Bruch reports that people she treats for eating disorders usually have faulty hunger awareness.

SOURCES OF FAULTY HUNGER AWARENESS

Theory #1

Dr. Bruch suggests that hunger awareness develops in infancy through a repeated chain of events. We feel uncomfortable because we're hungry, we cry, we're fed, and we feel better because our hunger has been sated. After a while we make the connection: "Those unpleasant sensations go away when I eat . . . here they are again so I must need to eat." Much later, when we learn to talk, those sensations are labeled hunger.[1]

Dr. Bruch suggests that some people de-velop faulty hunger awareness because their parents respond to their needs inappropriately. For example, suppose an infant cries because she needs to be cuddled, and the parent offers her a bottle or breast. If the infant refuses to eat and the parent repeatedly responds by putting her down, the infant will learn to eat in response to loneliness. This scenario may be repeated for many kinds of distress other than hunger if the parents generally respond to crying with feeding. The infant not only learns to eat in response to all kinds of distress, but also fails to differentiate among her needs.

Dr. Bruch contends that one of the causes of obesity is faulty hunger awareness developed in infancy. This may be true; however, as explained in Chapter 2, many fat people are fat because they are genetically designed to be fat (not because they eat too much). Therefore, this theory is often inapplicable.

Theory #2

Most of the people in my workshops enjoyed effortlessly accurate hunger awareness throughout childhood. Thus, assuming faulty hunger awareness is a symptom of eating disorders, it seems that we can develop faulty hunger awareness in childhood, in adolescence, or, most likely, at any age.

During infancy certain pleasant feelings tend to accompany feeding: physical comfort and warmth, close contact with another human being, and the feeling of being unconditionally loved and cared for. According to the principles of classical conditioning, eating should automatically trigger the same pleasant feelings of comfort, safety, and being loved and cared for even though the original cause of those feelings (contact with the parent) is missing. Consequently, if we're lonely, eating may trigger the wonderful, needed feelings of contact and being loved. If we're anxious or upset, eating may provide a calming, soothing effect. Thus, we may experience eating as a pacifier and comforter not only because eating is a sensual pleasure, but because it triggers a chain of positive feelings.

If eating has this powerful effect on us, then all kinds of negative feelings can become confused with hunger. When eating makes us feel better—not because we needed nourishment but because we needed nurturing—then we can logically, yet mistakenly, conclude that we were hungry.

Fatigue and other forms of physical discomfort might also be habitually mistaken for hunger because eating provides some relief. Fatigue can be caused by a need for sleep or mental rest and relaxation, or it can be caused by a need to eat. I can remember being incredibly tired as I was "pulling an all-nighter," and eating to gain energy. My fatigue was, without a doubt, caused by a need for sleep, but eating nonetheless helped me stay awake. We can get into the habit of interpreting and responding to a need for sleep as a need for food partly because eating can decrease fatigue and, thereby, reinforce our error.

So many people report that times of stress lead to overeating and weight gain that the connection is unquestionable. Consequently, many people assume that this type of "food abuse" is a major *cause* of chronic weight problems. "Excess weight" is said to be a mere symptom of underlying problems. Many people have been encouraged to

search for these underlying problems and to learn to cope with them differently.

This theory seems promising because it fits in with many psychologists' beliefs about learning and conditioning, as well as with common beliefs about the causes of overeating. However, it rests on the assumption that "weight problems" are usually caused by overeating. Since this is false, faulty hunger awareness (and consequent eating in response to nonnutritional needs) is not likely to be a very common *cause* of weight problems or eating disorders.

Dangers of the Theories

Most people who are preoccupied with diet and weight blame themselves for their problems. Unfortunately, the above theories feed into their self-doubts and self-condemnation. They already suspect that they are "compulsive eaters"—the theories implicitly confirm these suspicions by describing reasons for it.

Imagine a young woman who has just lost fifteen pounds through a weight-loss diet. She is pleased because she looks the way she would like to look in a bathing suit. But she is also frustrated because she is becoming increasingly preoccupied with food. Every time she loses weight she finds it more difficult to avoid bingeing. She wonders what is wrong with her: why does she feel so hungry, sometimes even after a meal?

We know why: she has dieted herself down to below her setpoint. She is therefore experiencing the normal effects of being underfed and underweight. But she doesn't know that. Now suppose that she reads one or both of the above theories. She will come away thinking that she has learned the cause of her "excessive hunger" and "compulsive eating." But she hasn't. In fact, she has just been given another reason to doubt her body's very real and appropriate signals. "I was right," she's now thinking, "I'm not *really* hungry!"

An Alternative Cause of Faulty Hunger Awareness

Most people who are preoccupied with diet and weight have decided that hunger, regardless of its source, is not necessarily an acceptable reason to eat. They expect to gain weight if they always eat in response to hunger. Therefore, *their eating has become a series of conscious and painful decisions quite unrelated to hunger.* Meanwhile, their body hunger remains intact and often surfaces in strong, vengeful waves. They fight against these waves of hunger because *they want to control their diets with their minds and ignore their bodies.*

The wide selection of appetite suppressants now on the market attests to this attitude toward hunger. We live in a society that encourages people to ignore or "turn off" their hunger pangs in order to lose weight. Dieters who consider appetite suppressants the "cheater's" way to overcome hunger try to obliterate hunger with their minds.

The human mind is capable of controlling and ignoring hunger. Almost everyone has felt hungry at an inconvenient time and chosen to ignore it. When we are absorbed in activities, our hunger can fade into the background. Those who want to lose weight not only ignore their hunger, they "talk themselves out of feeling it." Is it at all surprising that so many of us have faulty hunger awareness? Not at all. We live in a society overflowing with dieters who see their hunger as a dangerous enemy, whose influence they need to escape. We strive for faulty hunger awareness, and we get it.

Demon Hunger

Most of us have experienced hunger that we wanted to ignore and deny, but couldn't and didn't. We don't understand where this kind of hunger is coming from. We think it shouldn't be so strong; or it shouldn't have come on so soon after eating; or it shouldn't exist at this time of day or night; or worse yet, we should feel stuffed, not hungry. We tell ourselves not to trust our hunger. Experiences of insatiability and strong cravings for "bad" foods are especially difficult to understand. We ignore the possibility that we could be experiencing body hunger and decide our appetite is *irrational mind hunger.* We consider ourselves irrational for feeling it and responding to it.

Watching ourselves eat when we feel desperate to eat, yet desperate to stop eating, is a horrifying experience. We assume that the voice of the inner dieter is rational, and that the hungry voice is evil and irrational. We are horrified when hunger wins. I call this overpowering hunger "demon hunger," because many people feel it possesses them like a starving, demoniac entity.

Virtually everyone who reduces her weight through prolonged undereating experiences demon hunger. The wrestlers and rowers (described in Chapter 2) who cut weight experienced and responded to demon hunger after weekly competitions, and for months after the season ended. Dr. Keys's experimentally underfed men experienced demon hunger during the latter part of the experiment and during refeeding. Both groups' hunger and eating were normal and unconflicted until they restricted their diets and lost weight. Their demon hunger was caused by being underfed and underweight.

Anorexics and bulimics also experience demon hunger. Is their demon hunger a form of body hunger or mind hunger? Since anorexics are literally starving to death, their demon hunger is certainly body hunger. Most bulimics are malnourished as a result of purging (and usually poor eating) and may be below their setpoint weights. Thus, bulimics' demon hunger is also likely to be body hunger.

Many chronic dieters experience demon hunger as well. Is *their* demon hunger from a different source? Is it "just psychological"? Some chronic dieters attempt to maintain very low weights, which obviously lead to physiological demon hunger. The controversy begins when we consider chronic dieters who are obese, or "slightly overweight," or of average weight. Many of these people experience demon hunger as well. If setpoint theory is correct, then different people's bodies are genetically predisposed to have different percentages of body fat. A person can look overweight, yet *be underweight* and undernourished, and therefore experience the same demon hunger that anorexics, bulimics, and thin chronic dieters experience.

Regardless of how intense demon hunger becomes, it is *possible* to control food intake. We can deny our bodies carbohydrates no matter how much they scream with need, and we can deny ourselves food until we die of starvation. If this were not so, political protesters and anorexics would not be able to starve themselves to death. In order to deny demon hunger, however, we must have tremendous self-destructive conviction. We must believe that starvation is somehow essential—that unless we persist, we are in some way doomed. Once we are that desperate, all kinds of irrational mind games and intricate methods of avoiding "unwanted calories" become possible. Our minds are so powerful that we are capable of almost anything, including profound self-deception.

Fooling Ourselves Through Mind Games

I played many intricate mind games to lose weight. First, I consciously rejected my previous assumption (and years of proof) that weight control required constant self-deprivation. I decided that I would eat whatever I wanted, whenever I wanted, but would *never* eat unless I *really* wanted to. Every time I was about to eat something, no matter what it was, no matter how long it had been since I last ate, and regardless of whether it was a snack or a meal, I would ask myself, "Do I *really* want this? Am I going to feel *really* deprived and unhappy without it?" And more often than not, I decided that my desire to eat wasn't *really* strong enough. I didn't eat much, lost weight very rapidly, yet was convinced that I wasn't depriving myself. In reality, I was starving.

I used another mind game to redefine what it meant to be filled and to be hungry. I dreaded feeling filled because it meant that I didn't need to (and therefore "shouldn't") eat any more. I dreaded this because my long history of self-deprivation had taught me to despise and fear any feeling that I "shouldn't eat." I wanted to pretend that at *every* given moment I was totally free and allowed to eat. I liked to feel hungry—at least a little hungry—*all the time.* Hunger became a reassuring feeling rather than an uncomfortable feeling, and satiation became an uncomfortable feeling, rather than a feeling of satisfaction. Quite a complicated trick just to avoid eating!

I lived on a semistarvation diet for almost two years. Meanwhile, I was totally convinced that I was not dieting, that I was not suffering from constant hunger and deprivation, and that my diet/weight problems were permanently solved. I refused to define my hunger as real hunger unless I was about to eat a small amount that I had decided I really wanted and needed. When I *decided* I had had enough to eat, I also decided to *feel* that I had had enough to eat. "Why," I was forced to wonder, "do I dream about food?" But I was very good at ignoring these dreams and other symptoms of semistarvation. I didn't want to admit that I still had problems with diet and weight.

Most people who are preoccupied with diet and weight play a thousand mind games like these. If you have a long history of diet/weight conflicts, then your hunger awareness has probably been heightened through frequent self-analysis and attempts to draw lines between body hunger and mind hunger; however, you have fought against—and thereby abused and distorted—your hunger awareness as well.

Your hunger awareness is different from nondieters' hunger awareness in that you *think about* hunger and try to destroy it, while nondieters simply respond to it. Your *ability* to identify hunger is not the primary problem. The way you choose to deal with hunger, food, and eating is the problem.

DIETERS' MIND-SET

As we struggle with prolonged, self-imposed dietary restrictions, we develop a rigid and predictable way of thinking about our eating and ourselves. I call this way of thinking "dieters' mind-set" because it is a direct result of restrictive dieting.

When we have dieters' mind-set, dietary self-deprivation and weight control are a way of life. After months or years of continuous self-deprivation, it seems we never stop wanting to eat foods we "shouldn't" eat. We believe that tremendous willpower is necessary to prevent us from mis-eating at every opportunity. We begin to skip the internal question "Do I want to eat X?" and move directly to "Can I resist eating X?"

Chronic dieters refer to any eating we are trying to avoid as "bad" eating. We define certain foods and excessive amounts of food as "bad." We base these definitions on beliefs about what is "fattening" according to our latest "expert." Since most experts disagree, almost any food can be labeled "bad."

For instance, one diet book promotes foods high in fat and protein and low in carbohydrates.[2] Another argues that fat and sugar are the dieter's worst enemies and that carbohydrates should be the primary ingredients of our diets.[3] A third asserts that *all* foods are okay as long as they are eaten in the right combinations![4] "Experts" produce countless definitions of "good" and "bad" eating.

In reality, "bad" eating simply refers to *disallowed* eating. What we accept as "good" and "bad" is often misguided and unreasonable. Anorexics, for instance, continually define the food they so desperately need as "bad." Anyone who is desperate to lose weight—anorexic or not—is likely to diet in an unhealthy way. Whatever is considered "bad" I call "disallowed," in order to emphasize that our definitions are neither consistent nor, in most cases, rational.

Dieters' mind-set guarantees an unsatisfying and painful relationship with food. Consider what happens when we ask ourselves: "Can I resist eating this disallowed food (X)?" We may decide not to eat X or anything else. Consequently, we will feel proud of our willpower and relieved that we resisted temptation. But we may also feel deprived, annoyed, and hungry. Worse yet, we will become preoccupied with thoughts of when and what food we *will* allow ourselves. In short, it's a dismal and unsatisfying option.

We may decide to eat allowed food Y instead of disallowed food X. Again, we may feel proud and relieved; however, this solution is also less than satisfying. Often it seems that nothing but food X, or a similar food, will satisfy our hunger. For instance, suppose we want a piece of bread or some other carbohydrate but have disallowed carbohydrates. We may try to still our craving with low-fat cottage cheese, or some other allowed food. However, even if we consume a lot of allowed food, we can continue to crave (and need!) carbohydrates. We are left feeling dissatisfied. We may even eat X after failing to satisfy ourselves with allowed food, and this experience reinforces the belief that our hunger is irrational and harmful. Again, it's a less than satisfying option.

A third possibility is that we eat food X despite our determination to resist it. We feel guilty for betraying our convictions. We see ourselves as out of control and "bad." We may even define the entire day as "bad." We are likely to begin thinking about how we are going to "make up for it." Our choice to eat what we wanted should have been satisfying. Instead, any satisfaction is overshadowed, if not destroyed, by regret, guilt, and dread of the supposed consequences. Once again—a painful option.

No one enjoys living with dieters' mind-set. However, we cling to it in the hope that this restrictive way of thinking and eating will promote weight control. Does dieters' mind-set promote weight control? Sometimes. But it usually has the opposite effect.

Dieters' mind-set consists of self-imposed pressure not to eat, and it assumes a constant desire to eat in a fattening way. When we assume that we always want to eat, we give up the best and most pleasant reason for not eating—not wanting to eat. In addition, we punish ourselves for disallowed eating. The rationale is this: if I punish myself, I will pay for my "bad" eating, and I will learn to curb my appetite. In practice, however, this doesn't work. Punishing ourselves for disallowed eating often leads to further disallowed eating.

Why? First, because guilt, self-disgust, recrimination, and other forms of self-punishment make us feel bad, and when we feel bad we need and want to comfort ourselves. One of the ways we have learned to

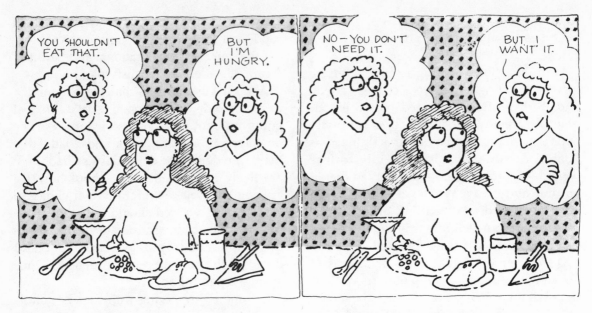

comfort ourselves is by eating delicious food.

Second, if we treat ourselves as misbehaved children or convicts, then we begin to feel like we are misbehaved children or convicts. How do children and convicts feel? *They feel a lack of control over their own lives, and they yearn for self-determination and freedom.* They are expected to obey and "answer to" authority figures, and, in general, they respond with anger, outrage, and *rebellion.*

Third, if we define ourselves or our day as "bad" because we fail to control our eating, we set ourselves up for further disallowed eating. Once we have defined ourselves as "bad" or "out of control," we feel that, by definition, we will continue to eat in a disallowed way. If we also define the day as "bad," then it feels as though we have "nothing more to lose by going all the way." (We'll make up for it tomorrow by being really "good"—maybe we'll fast. . . .)

Fourth, and perhaps most compelling, is the pull to eat when we are anticipating future deprivation. Whenever we plan to go hungry, our desire to eat increases automatically. This is not an irrational reaction. Everyone who knows of an approaching famine instinctually wants to "store up" in preparation.

If we feel that we must continually restrict our food intake, we are set up for endless cycles of hated self-deprivation and hated "loss of control." Diets are like jails that every normal human being would want to escape. Once we escape, we want to stay out as long as possible and make the best of it. Any day, any hour, we know that we may return to jail. In this way, the specter of past and future deprivation encourages disallowed eating. Both physically and psychologically, the natural preparation for and reaction to food deprivation is bingeing.

In summary, long-term food restrictions can cause more disallowed eating than would otherwise occur because they lead to (a) food preoccupation, (b) the assumption

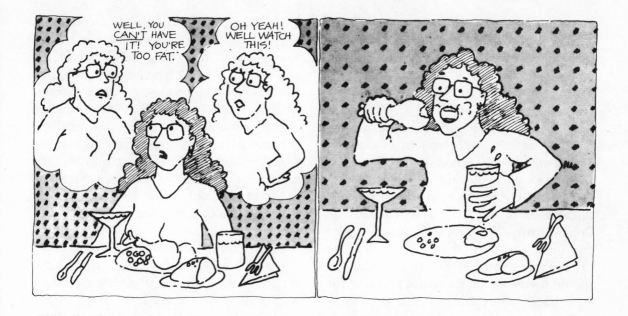

that we want disallowed food, (c) guilt, which leads to unhappiness, which in turn leads to comforting disallowed eating, (d) feelings of anger and rebellion against the authoritative "dieter," (e) self-fulfilling definitions of ourselves and the day as "bad," and (f) thoughts, plans, and fears about future deprivation that increase our desires to "eat while we can." Thus *dieters' mind-set leads to a painful relationship with food without promoting diet or weight control.*

A Few Big Meals Versus Many Small Meals

Even when dieters' mind-set does not lead to greater food intake (overall), it almost always leads to "bunching up" of food intake. In other words, it leads to periods of very little eating and periods of hearty eating.

What are the physiological effects of this eating pattern? We know that undereating leads to lower metabolic rates. Your body tries to adjust and "make do" with what you give it without depleting fat stores any more than necessary. When you eat very little, your body reacts defensively. What happens when, suddenly, you eat a lot more than usual? Your body has been well prepared to turn food into body fat because it has learned to get by on very little.

So the same amount of food can lead to different amounts of weight gain or loss, depending on when it is eaten. If you are in the habit of alternating between low-calorie diets and binges, you are promoting a higher weight than you would promote by eating the same amount of food spread out more evenly. Furthermore, if you tend to eat little or nothing during the day and a lot at night (a very common pattern among dieters), you are promoting a higher weight than if you were to eat three normal meals per day. Thus

Learning to Eat Spontaneously

dieters' mind-set leads to eating patterns that promote higher, rather than lower, weights.

Two Experiences of Disallowed Eating

Two examples of disallowed eating and the resulting feelings and behavior will illustrate dieters' mind-set in action.

Suppose you have just started to eat a bowl of ice cream. As hard as you try, you cannot seem to justify this disallowed eating. Consequently, you feel increasingly guilty and upset—you are "bad." The more you eat, the worse you feel. You believe that you should not be eating ice cream and that the logical and correct thing to do is *stop* eating it. At the same time, you feel increasingly frantic to continue eating. It tastes good, and you have a vague and dreadful feeling that your next ice cream is a millennium away.

Why are so many of us capable of becoming frantic over a bowl of ice cream? Partly because we should not eat ice cream, according to our dietary rules. It is "too fattening" and, therefore, the longer we can resist its wonderful creamy sweetness, the better. We may even feel that we should never eat ice cream again. In theory, this is the only way to be completely "good." Most of us do not consider this drastic, eternal deprivation a real possibility; however, we know that we will again promise ourselves to "be good." Not surprisingly, we feel compelled to eat and enjoy while we can.

Another common conflict may arise as we approach the end of a meal or snack. The usual goal is to stop eating after we have consumed a meager, allowed amount of food. Part of dieters' mind-set can make this a very painful task. Many of us do not allow snacking and skip meals whenever we can manage it. We want to eat very sparsely. But because it is difficult to avoid overeating, we want to make up for past or future excesses whenever possible. The fewer times we eat, the less often we have to deal with food and risk mis-eating (most people find it much easier to abstain than to eat a little). The fewer times we eat, the more we can afford to eat at one sitting; the less we eat now, the more we can afford to eat later. Sound familiar?

One of the many problems with this policy is that the end of every meal or snack becomes the beginning of an undetermined period of deprivation. We know from experience that the next time we want something to eat, we are likely to deny ourselves, or at least try to deny ourselves. Consequently, the fear and dread of future hunger, as well as (in some cases) insatiability caused by previous deprivation, can lead to a strong desire to prolong meals.

Many dieters report that the sight of their empty plates causes feelings of panic and a powerful longing to refill them before the meal ends.[5] We feel upset if we have just eaten but are unsatisfied. We do not want to face the painful decision of whether or not to stop eating despite our hunger. We rarely understand the source of this panic, so we explain it by labeling ourselves "pigs" or "compulsive overeaters." Our diets leave us hungry and unsatisfied, and therefore we want to eat more. We are not absurdly greedy. We are merely attempting to meet our basic needs.

Compulsive Eating

We need to distinguish between disallowed eating and "losing control" or "compulsive eating." If we *decide* to eat a disallowed food because we are not willing to deny ourselves, that is disallowed eating. We are in control, we simply choose to eat something disallowed. Compulsive eating, on the other hand, is eating with the feeling that we can't stop ourselves. We don't want to keep eating, but we have lost control. All compulsive eating is disallowed eating; however, not all disallowed eating is compulsive.

When does disallowed eating become compulsive eating? First, recall that when we eat disallowed food, we "lose" an internal battle between our desire to deny ourselves and our desire to eat. (I say "lose" because we define our dietary restrictions as rational, and our hunger as "the enemy.") While eating, we think about the weight we expect to gain, and are therefore upset by our behavior. We feel that by eating we are doing an irrational and self-destructive thing. We want to restrict our eating, but we are not doing so. We cannot accept blatantly irrational behavior. Consequently, we try to come up with an explanation.

Suppose that we feel extremely unhappy and desperate. We might reason that we cannot bear to increase our unhappiness and desperation by starving ourselves. Or suppose our relatives look hurt because we do not seem to appreciate their food. We might decide that our "diets" are less important than their feelings. An endless number of justifications are possible. If, however, we cannot justify and rationalize our disallowed eating (but nonetheless continue to eat), our minds can refuse to take part in our irrational behavior. We can begin to eat without thinking about it. We avoid awareness of how much or exactly what we are eating, and eat quickly. We feel as though at any moment we may be forced to stop eating. How forced? Anything that would make us fully conscious of ourselves might force us to re-evaluate what we're doing and consider other options.

This is compulsive eating or losing control: we feel incapable of controlling our eating because we cannot stop or control behavior we have refused to acknowledge as our own.

Why do we feel compelled to do something we are determined not to do? Most of us reach a point at which diet and weight control seem so important that no reason is acceptable. At the same time, our demon hunger can become so intense that the internal battle is unbearable. The source of this hunger is physiological need combined with desperation to end the torture of habitual self-denial; however, we experience it as an irrational force that rises from within.

Barriers Along the Road to Freedom

Dieters' mind-set is very difficult to escape for at least four reasons. First, if a physiological conflict remains, then the psychological conflict, and our defenses for dealing with it, will also remain. Many of us choose goal weights below our bodies' setpoints; consequently, we enter a battle between our bodies' strong and endless needs and our attempts to become and remain thin. Dieters' mind-set is a natural and logical way to think if we are continually trying to deny our bodies' powerful demands. We accept the constant pain of hunger and self-deprivation because that is the true price of becoming and remaining underweight.

The second reason why dieters' mind-set is difficult to destroy is that our attitudes toward hunger produce poor hunger awareness. We become accustomed to fighting and denying hunger and, simultaneously, afraid to feel and respond to it. We choose to control our eating on the basis of "reason," rather than accepting hunger as a cue for eating. Paying attention to our hunger seems unpredictable, undisciplined, and dangerous: we want "too much"; we want the "wrong" things; we can't trust ourselves.

The third and closely related difficulty is that memories of long-term deprivation and intense conflict fade slowly and may never disappear. After years of self-deprivation, it is difficult to completely believe that we are never going to starve ourselves again. We expect yet another bout of self-deprivation to be lurking around the next corner. (Which is natural until we learn to accept and appreciate our bodies.) This fear and dread of future deprivation, along with memories of past deprivation, are major constituents and causes of dieters' mind-set. Neither will fade unless we are convinced that our days of self-deprivation are over.

Even some of the postseason wrestlers and rowers who knew that they could relax and return to their normal eating patterns (until next year) found it difficult to resume the completely carefree eating they enjoyed before cutting weight. Some reported that their experiences of self-deprivation led to excessive eating off-season. Recovered anorexics also complain of lingering problems. In fact, the vast majority of recovered anorexics suffer from painful conflicts regarding diet and weight on a daily basis.

The fourth source of support for dieters' mind-set is widespread cultural images and public opinion. The attitudes of friends and relatives encourage dieters' mind-set. Preoccupation with appearance and weight-loss dieting are widely respected. Friends and relatives often applaud dietary restrictions and attitudes that are an integral part of dieters' mind-set. The media, of course, also reinforce dieters' mind-set through pressure to control diet/weight and the attitude that "it isn't easy, but you can do it." Thus, dieters' mind-set is generally considered "normal" and "good," at least until it becomes a central symptom of an eating disorder.

STEPS TOWARD SPONTANEOUS EATING

Dieters' mind-set is caused by long-term struggles to lose (and maintain) weight. It develops as you diet even if you are a "normal dieter." The longer you restrict your diet as part of a struggle for weight control, the more rigid dieters' mind-set becomes. Thus, dieters' mind-set develops along with your preoccupation, and later reinforces and maintains it.

Dieters' mind-set sometimes helps to enforce dietary restrictions. More often, however, it leads to more disallowed eating than would have occurred if you had not become a perpetual dieter. The defensive desires and behavior that result from chronic self-deprivation cause this irony. In any case, dieters' mind-set guarantees that eating is painful: it is "controlled" (less than desired), or it is "uncontrolled" (more than "allowed"). You are either in the weight reduction jail, or you have temporarily escaped and are "going wild" while you can.

In order to gain freedom from your diet/weight obsession, you need to gain freedom from dieters' mind-set. You must replace dieters' mind-set with a different way of thinking about, and coping with, hunger and food. In other words, you must stop depriving yourself and learn to eat spontaneously on a daily basis.

You may think that you already know how to eat spontaneously, and that spontaneous eating is your enemy. This is extremely unlikely. Are you able to think about a delicious dessert, decide that you want to eat it, and do so *without arguing with yourself and without feeling guilty?* If not, then you have (temporarily) lost the ability to eat spontaneously. Spontaneous eating is eating in response to desire without internal conflict.

In order to eat spontaneously, you must try to eat without compulsion. In other words, *you must constantly reassure yourself that you never have to eat anything you don't want, and that you never have to deprive yourself of something you do want.* At first (and perhaps for a long time) this will be very difficult to do. You will be tempted to return to the familiar "safety" of compulsive dieting and eating. When that temptation arises, remind yourself that down that path lies chronic dieting, preoccupation, and all the pain and unhappiness associated with it. Try to focus on how much you can enjoy what you eat, and to eat the exact foods and amounts you will most enjoy.

Once you have attained freedom from diet/weight conflict, you can go back to eating things you don't really want in order to be polite now and then. You can eliminate some or all of the "unhealthy elements" from your diet. In short, you can eat in whatever way you choose. In order to gain freedom from preoccupation, however, you need first to eat without depriving yourself of anything you want, and not eat when you don't feel like it.

As you focus on your desires and attempt to fulfill them noncompulsively, try to maintain your physical comfort. It is very unpleasant to feel *ravenously* hungry, and it is at least as unpleasant to feel totally "stuffed." Do your best to avoid these feelings. At the same time, do not feel guilty if you fail to maintain your physical comfort. People who are coming off restrictive diets often find that they are unable to avoid food binges. Our bodies often demand compensation. This has been observed among people who have been restricting their diets for mere months. If you have been trying to restrict your diet, then understand that it is natural and normal, not crazy or horrible, for you to "go wild" for a while.

On the other hand, *don't assume* that you will need to binge. Some people never need to binge once they stop dieting because most of their suffering was based on dieters' mind-set. In other words, they assumed they wanted to eat too much, and they feared and dreaded future deprivation while they remained dieters; however, once these assumptions and fears were eliminated by becoming nondieters, their reactive need to binge disappeared.[6]

Here's another important rule to remember and follow: if you crave a certain food, then you must have and enjoy it free of guilt or regret regardless of what it is (unless it's unavailable). You must stop depriving yourself and learn to be proud of this sensible behavior. If you crave one food, don't try to fulfill your craving with a different, "better" food. You will not only have supported dieters' mind-set, reactive overeating, and diet/weight preoccupation, you will have robbed yourself of the most enjoyable eating experience in existence—fulfilling a strong craving. Even the most delicious gourmet food, prepared by the greatest chef in the world, will not taste as good as a food for which you have spontaneously developed a craving. Appreciate and enjoy your cravings!

Most of the time, you will find that you don't crave anything in particular. You will be hungry and know that you want something to eat, but you won't have a *strong* preference. Whenever this happens, *try to choose nutritious foods.* Eat low-fat, low-sugar, low-salt foods rather than junk food. Choose brown rice, whole wheat bread, or baked potatoes over white rice, white bread, or french fries. Choose chicken or fish over red meat. And, as usual, do your best to eat the amount that makes you feel best: be sated but not stuffed.

Nutritious eating can go a long way toward making you feel good. Malnutrition, on the other hand, can increase your cravings for high-fat, high-sugar foods and make you feel rotten. It is not difficult to eat well (see Chapter 8). It *is* difficult to deprive yourself of food you need and want.

In *How to Lower Your Fat Thermostat,* Drs. Remington, Fisher, and Parent suggest that eating three meals a day on a regular basis helps dieters reconnect with hunger and sa-

tiation. At breakfast and lunch they recommend that you eat until satisfied but not completely full. At dinner, they recommend that you eat a nutritionally complete meal and that you eat more than at other meals—until you are completely sated. If you get hungry between meals, they recommend light snacks.

This advice is contrary to the popular notion that it is better for you to eat more during the day while you are active and burning lots of energy, and eat less in the evening when you are less active and soon to sleep. However, my own experience is that this "inverted triangle" pattern of eating during the day makes me less alert and less energetic during the day and leaves me hungry at night. In short, it doesn't *feel good* and it doesn't come naturally.

Years before I read Remington, Fisher, and Parent's work, I spontaneously developed exactly the eating pattern they described. As I struggled to reconnect with my hunger and satiation signals, I found myself eating light breakfasts and lunches and relatively heavy dinners (plus snacks). Furthermore, in workshops I have observed that those who skip meals, or avoid real meals completely, do not progress toward freedom from diet/weight conflict or develop spontaneous eating as quickly as those who eat three meals a day on a regular basis. In addition, chronic dieters who decide to eat three meals a day do not, as a rule, become heavier than those who eat fewer meals per day. If anything, the opposite is true.

Only you can decide the pattern of eating that best suits your needs. However, I recommend that you at least try out eating three meals a day for the following reasons:

1. It is more convenient. You can schedule meals into your day much like non-dieters and be more in sync with other people.

2. You can habitually eat meals and thereby spend less time worrying about when and if you're going to eat. You will therefore be less preoccupied with food.

3. Eating regular meals will keep you from getting *excessively* hungry, which will decrease the desire and tendency to binge as well as decrease food preoccupation prior to eating.

4. Eating regular meals will allow you to reexperience the natural pattern of hunger, satiation, gradually returning hunger, satiation, etc.

5. Eating regular meals, providing they do not include a lot of sugar, will make you feel more energetic, increase your tendency to move and burn more energy, help you be more productive, and, most important, help you enjoy life more fully.

Regardless of whether or not you ultimately choose to eat three meals a day, keep in mind the keys to spontaneous eating, which are listening and responding to hunger and satiation, meeting nutritional needs, and eating what you want without guilt.

Why is it so important to learn to eat spontaneously? What are we trying to accomplish? The primary goal is to overcome diet/weight conflict, but we must meet many intermediate goals on the way.

Your first goal is to enjoy eating. Most of us need to give ourselves permission to enjoy eating. We have come to fear and feel guilty for this enjoyment, and have thereby robbed ourselves of it. If we enjoy our food, then we will feel more comfortable and satisfied with our eating. We will no longer search for satisfaction through bingeing.

Your second goal is to end your preoccupation with food. Ultimately, food preoccupation leads to painful stuffing and starving, depression, anger, and frustration. Unfulfilled desires and needs to eat cause food preoccupation. If you eat whatever you want whenever you want, then you will soon (but not immediately) stop being preoccupied with food.

Your third goal is to end the battle between your mind and body by effortlessly maintaining a comfortable (setpoint) weight. If you have been struggling with your diet and weight since adolescence or earlier, you probably couldn't determine your setpoint in Chapter 2. The only way to determine your setpoint, then, is to stop struggling with your diet and weight. If the reactive symptoms of dieters' mind-set, coupled with intermittent reducing regimens, have been pushing your weight upward, then you will eventually come to rest at a lower weight through spontaneous eating. If, on the other hand, you have been struggling to stay under your setpoint weight, then you will eventually come to rest at this higher, healthier weight.

I know: the prospect of being "too fat" is scaring you to death. You're not alone. *Most* of us, in fact, would like to be thinner than our setpoints dictate, whether we have unusually high *or* unusually low setpoints. The only reassurance I can offer is that as you free yourself from dieters' mind-set, ornamental body views, feelings of inefficacy,

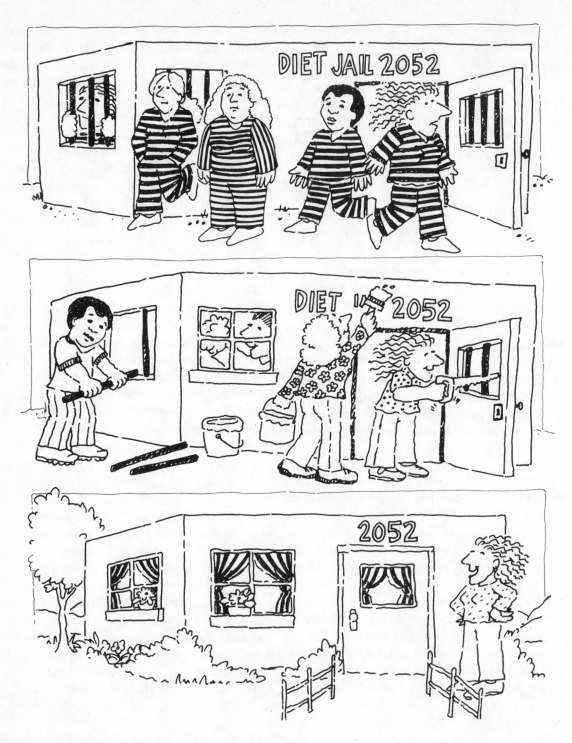

and lack of control, your body weight will matter to you less and less. Your weight will no longer dictate your level of self-esteem, nor will it determine your physical comfort and satisfaction. It's hard to believe, but living at your active setpoint weight (the weight your body defends when you are exercising regularly) *will feel good* and right! You will no longer be plagued by demon hunger, and you will be more energetic and strong. In short, you and your body will finally be at peace with each other. You will have come home.

When you begin to retrain yourself to eat spontaneously, you may feel *more* preoccupied with food at first. Try to be patient with yourself. You've probably spent years—perhaps your whole life—practicing and learning to eat and think like a chronic dieter. It will take consistent, deliberate work to relearn to eat without conflict or compulsion.

When I stopped restricting my diet and began to gain weight, I fought my anxiety by reassuring myself that I could always diet back down to my previous weight. I knew that this was a destructive thought—a cornerstone of dieters' mind-set—but my anxiety was sometimes so intense that I could not help thinking it. Every now and then I began to restrict my diet again because my anxiety was too great to bear. Gradually, however, I relearned to eat spontaneously. Do not think that if you occasionally slip back into your old ways, all progress has been lost. These periods of compulsively controlled or uncontrolled eating can actually reinforce your understanding of the damaging effects and help you progress toward freedom.

Ideally, every reader would pause right now and think: "Well, that's it. I'm never going on a weight-loss diet again. I'm never again going to deny myself food I really want. It's over." If you can simply make that decision, and thereby be rid of dieters' mind-set and diet/weight conflict—I congratulate you. Unfortunately, most of you will find it very hard to commit yourselves to this decision. You will have to start smaller and gradually chop away at your dieters' mind-set and dieting behavior.

Relearning to eat spontaneously can be a long and difficult process. Anxiety—caused by your fear of gaining weight—will be your greatest challenge. That anxiety leads to eating more than you really want, eating less than you really want, and planning future deprivation and weight loss. Thus *anxiety pushes you toward action that is anxiety-reducing but ultimately destructive.* You will need to respond to anxiety in a different way.

How? Try using these three steps:

1. Accept the anxiety as your own and allow yourself to experience it fully.

2. Acknowledge the destructive nature of the anxiety.

3. Let go of it—allow it to pass by without being manipulated and harmed by it.

Step #1: Allow Yourself to Experience It Fully

In order to deal with a self-destructive thought, feeling, or action, we need to accept it as our own and allow ourselves to experience it fully *without judging* it or ourselves.

Most of us have been taught to deal with unpleasant feelings such as anxiety, disappointment, and sadness by denying their existence. We are supposed to push negative thoughts and feelings out of our minds and pretend that everything is fine. In theory, this does away with the problem; in reality, this usually encourages the problem to remain and grow within us.

We have also been taught to deal with destructive actions by punishing ourselves and then forcing ourselves to behave differently. Thus, we have learned to treat ourselves as bad children who need to be forcibly changed by a stern parent. This, too, tends to be ineffective. What we really want to do and what we tell ourselves to do seem to be at odds; consequently, we do not change.

Ultimately, we want to let go of self-destructive thoughts, feelings, and actions; however, *we cannot let go of anything we refuse to face and acknowledge as our own*. The first step toward freedom, therefore, is to fully experience and accept whatever thought, feeling, or action is bothering us. Only *after* doing this will we be able to understand it and let go of it.

Step #2: Understand and Acknowledge Its Nature

Next we need to understand how the thought, feeling, or action is affecting us. Is it something we enjoy or benefit from in some way? How does it hurt us? In what way is it rational, and in what way is it irrational? Overall, is it self-supportive or self-destructive? In conclusion, would we like to keep it, or would we rather let go of it?

We need to evaluate the problematic thought, feeling, or action—not as "good" or "bad," but as something we enjoy and want, or as something we do not enjoy or want. However, *we must not judge ourselves*. Rather than thinking, "That thought (feeling or action) is irrational and self-destructive—what in the world is wrong with me?" we need to think, "That thought (feeling or action) is hurting me a lot more than it's helping me. I think I'd rather let go of it."

Step #3: Let Go of It When You Can

We have now done the groundwork for letting go; however, we still have to resist the temptation to *push* it away. Our instinct is to perform some kind of thought-ectomy, feeling-ectomy, or action-ectomy—to somehow cut it out of ourselves and thereby destroy it. If we truly want to be good to ourselves, heal ourselves, and grow, then we need to be patient. We need to change when we're ready and not push ourselves too hard. When we are truly ready to let go of a recurring thought, feeling, or action, we will not need to push it away, "cut it out," or "force ourselves"; we will simply let go of it—naturally choose peace of mind and greater satisfaction over struggle and dissatisfaction.

In Frank Herbert's science fiction epic *Dune*, certain characters cope with their fear by reciting a "Litany Against Fear." Whenever they become afraid, they say to themselves: "I must not fear. Fear is the mind-killer. Fear is the little-death that brings total obliteration. I will face my fear. I will permit it to pass over me and through me. And when it has gone past I will turn the inner eye to see its path. Where the fear has gone there will be nothing. Only I will remain."[7] I like this litany because it points to the steps that can help us let go of anxiety and fear. Just reading it is soothing. It encourages us to feel our inner strength—to recognize our infinite ability to cope and act wisely.

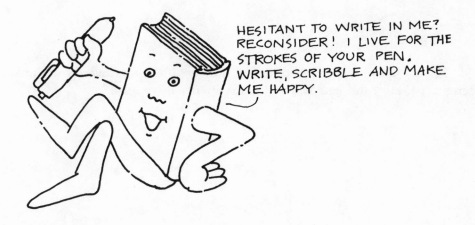

PERSONAL QUESTIONS:
FROM DIETER'S MIND-SET TO SPONTANEOUS EATING

1. Do you consider your hunger an enemy, a friend, or neither? Why?

2. Was there a time when you would have answered question 1 differently? If so, when and why did the change occur?

3. Have you ever experienced demon hunger? If so, what were you thinking during the experience(s)? How did you explain the experience to yourself?

4. If you experience demon hunger or something similar, do you think it is physically or psychologically induced (or both)? Are you sure of your answer? How could you test your answer?

5. Do you suffer from dieters' mind-set? If so, to what extent? Describe the way you think about your hunger, your eating, etc.

6. How does dieters' mind-set seem to help and hurt you?

7. Review the causes of reactive "overeating" (p. 77). Has dieters' mind-set ever led you to eat a lot? Overall, do you think that your mind-set leads you to eat more or less than is best for you?

8. Describe the way you thought about and dealt with your eating and weight before you developed dieters' mind-set. Would you like to be able to return to that way of thinking and eating?

9. How might replacing dieters' mind-set and chronic dieting with spontaneous eating help you? Make a list of all the benefits.

BENEFITS OF SPONTANEOUS EATING

10. List specific changes you can make (in attitude and/or behavior) that will undermine your dieters' mind-set and promote spontaneous eating.

TO UNDERMINE DIETERS' MIND-SET AND PROMOTE SPONTANEOUS EATING

11. What resources do you have to help you achieve these goals?

12. What will your challenges be? What will oppose your efforts?

13. What changes can you make right away that will lead toward your goals?

5

LEARNING TO LOVE OURSELVES

We all need to feel good about ourselves. We need to know that we are capable, loving, loved, respected, and worthy of other people's love and respect. We have to live with ourselves at all times; consequently, we cannot be happy unless we like ourselves. Our need for positive self-esteem is almost as compelling as our need for food and shelter. When our self-esteem is at risk, we naturally feel driven to do everything in our power to protect it.

If you are preoccupied with diet and weight, then your *self-esteem is probably strongly affected by diet/weight control:* when you control your diet and weight, you feel better about yourself; when you fail to control your diet and weight, you feel bad about yourself. As long as your self-esteem is tied up with diet/weight control, you will not be able to let go of dieters' mind-set, dieters' behavior, or your preoccupation. Your desperate need for positive self-esteem will drive you endlessly.

How can you disassociate your self-esteem from diet/weight control? We have already looked at two ways. First, by letting go of your *fattism* and opposing it in the world. Second, by letting go of your judgmental stance regarding food and eating. These changes are powerful, but they are only partial solutions to the problem.

Most of you have latched on to diet/weight control as a basis for self-improvement and, thus, as a potential source of positive self-esteem. Right now, diet/weight preoccupation is one of the "materials" that form the foundation of your self-esteem—a foundation that is very unstable. If you simply get rid of that "material" by letting go of your preoccupation, what will be left? Probably the very low self-esteem that exists now, minus some of your most powerful methods of coping with it (your focus on diet and weight as "the problem"). You cannot simply get rid of your preoccupation. You need to *replace* it with something else—something that will support instead of destroy your ability to live happily.

When I suggest to chronic dieters that they need to learn to accept and appreciate themselves as they are, someone usually responds: "But I don't want to accept myself as I am. I'm too fat. I don't like myself like this. I *shouldn't* like myself like this!" Clearly, my suggestion hits home. The reaction is pure terror.

We have been taught that personal progress comes from hating our shortcomings and *therefore* working to overcome them. We think that if we accept ourselves as we are, we will stop progressing. Misdirected by that lesson and fueled by fear, we refuse to appreciate our true value. We miss the fact that *we can accept and appreciate ourselves AND work toward desirable change.*

What will really happen if you learn to feel good about yourself exactly as you are? Will you say, "Phew! I've arrived. Now I don't have to work on anything anymore. I can stay just like this"? Of course not. The more we like ourselves, the more easily we change and grow. When we have a base of security, we feel confident and able to tackle challenges. Self-condemnation, fear of failure, and unhappiness go hand in hand. They hold us back far more than they push us forward.

The first two steps toward healthier self-esteem are (a) recognizing that you need to feel better about yourself, and (b) realizing that it would be helpful and sensible to feel good about yourself *exactly as you are*—that *you can begin to feel better about yourself right now on an unconditional basis.*

"Unconditional! But that's impossible!" people often say. "How I feel about myself depends on what I do, how I look, and whether or not people like me. I can't like

myself unconditionally." I answer with this question: "Can you *dislike* yourself unconditionally?" I'll bet that many of you do. I know that I did.

We tend to assume that self-esteem is determined by what we accomplish: attractiveness, popularity, career achievement, athletic achievement, academic achievement. This seems logical, but it is not true. *Many people who have virtually everything going for them nonetheless suffer from low self-esteem*, while others who have achieved little (according to our culture's values) sometimes enjoy positive self-esteem. We can hate ourselves without knowing why, and we can think we like ourselves, yet consistently reveal that we don't. If self-esteem were a simple reflection of our merits (versus shortcomings), this would not be possible.

You *can* like and accept yourself unconditionally. What does that mean? It means that your bottom line can be self-acceptance, appreciation, and understanding no matter what happens. Some use religion as the starting point for developing positive self-esteem: If God created you and loves you regardless of your weaknesses and mistakes, then you are always worthy and valuable in an absolute and unconditional way. You do not have to believe in God, however, to develop unconditional self-acceptance. All you have to do is change your assumptions and attitudes and begin to see yourself through different lenses—clear lenses instead of dark ones.

Within each of us is a warm and loving person. That is what we all are: beautiful, loving, absolutely lovable people. We may, for many different reasons, behave otherwise. But we can't change what's deep inside, and we are forever longing to behave like our true selves. We all want to be happy, and since the only way to be happy is to be that warm and loving person, we all wish to be so. When we are not acting as our true selves, that is just a reflection of the pain and fear (from the past and present) that darken our view of the world, other people, and ourselves. In every moment we do the best we can, and we need and deserve encouragement and appreciation.

Many of us have grown up amidst warnings about conceit and selfishness. Some of us have been told that self-love is a sin. Humility is admired. Suffering is respected. As a result, we end up valuing self-effacement, self-hatred, suffering, and guilt.

Imagine that you and your friend Sally are going to have dinner together. When you meet, Sally says, "You look great."

"Are you kidding?" you respond. "*I* don't think so."

She insists that you look beautiful. You thank her, but add that you feel ugly. The subject changes.

Why do we feel ugly? Why do we sidestep and contradict compliments? Why do we see and present ourselves in a negative way? We do not allow ourselves self-love. Some convoluted logic tells us that it is "good" to lack pride ("Pride goeth before a fall," you know), and to slight ourselves whenever we get the chance. Some convoluted logic tells us that suffering makes us good. Is this productive? Is it good for the world? Do people behave more morally from a basis of self-effacement and self-hatred? I think not.

If you feel good about yourself, you will be more likely to behave morally. If you like yourself and are good to yourself, you will be more likely to appreciate and be good to others, and vice versa. Furthermore, if you make a mistake, or if you fail to do something very important to you, nothing positive will be accomplished by hating yourself for it. We do not have to feel guilty and bad about ourselves in order to learn from mistakes. In fact, guilt and self-recrimination make it *harder* to respond to mistakes in a constructive way.

I am not saying that you should never feel bad—that is not an option for any human being. I *am* saying that you can value pride and unconditional self-respect and try to avoid self-condemnation. You deserve to feel good about yourself. You deserve to be happy. Believe in and strive for unconditional self-acceptance and appreciation.

Of course, this is not an easy or quick process. It took long years of training for you to learn to dislike yourself. It will take time and effort to let go of old assumptions and replace them with a positive outlook. Try to work toward real self-appreciation from as many angles as you can find.

SELF-ESTEEM, EFFICACY, AND CONFIDENCE

Dr. Nathaniel Branden argues that self-esteem cannot be stable and positive unless it is based upon self-efficacy.[1] Self-efficacy is an overall ability to survive in the world: to think, make decisions, and act in an effective and satisfying way. In other words, positive self-esteem requires that we feel able to live well—to enjoy life.

Do you lack self-efficacy? More important

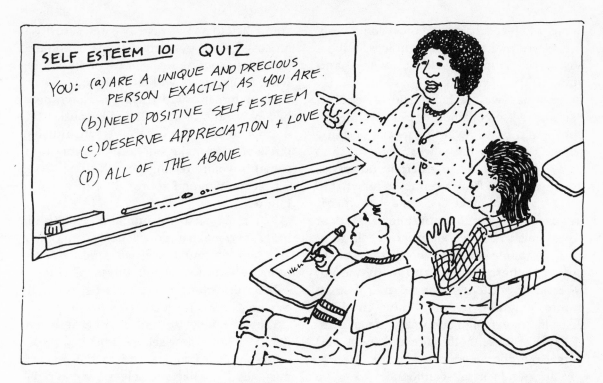

still: do you *feel* a lack of self-efficacy? Many people who are preoccupied with diet and weight are very strong and capable, yet *feel* ineffective. We may work very hard and accomplish a lot, yet suffer from chronic feelings of inadequacy. Others may see us as determined workers, while we feel like slaves who are constantly kept in line by our own anxiety.

A friend of mine, Jessica, illustrates this dichotomy. Jessica graduated cum laude from Harvard, did well in business school, and became a very successful consultant. One might expect that by this time Jessica would feel quite capable and successful, but she didn't. This incredibly intelligent and accomplished woman constantly belittled her achievements and herself. Deep inside she felt that she was doomed to fail socially

and professionally, and she spent her school years struggling with anorexia, bulimia, and chronic dieting. She worked very hard to avoid failure—and more than avoided it. Still, she remained haunted by the feeling that she was "barely scraping by."

I have seen this sort of problem over and over, first in myself, and then among my workshop participants and friends. We are so capable, yet we manage to *feel* like losers. Our achievements seem empty, and failure seems to be around every corner even when everything is going well. How can we be rational about everyone except ourselves?

We evaluate others through observation, but we evaluate ourselves from the inside out. We question our own actions: *why* do we do the things we do? Often, we feel *compelled* to action (by anxiety or other people).

Learning to Love Ourselves

In order to feel capable, we must confidently and freely make our own choices. Otherwise, we will feel selfless, weak, and vulnerable.

Every day we are faced with a series of decisions. We continually choose our actions. On a banal level this means deciding when to get up, what to wear, how much to study or work, how to entertain ourselves, whether or not to buy a certain item, what to eat. . . . We also make decisions that will affect us for longer periods of time: whether or not to finish high school or go to college or go to graduate school; what profession to pursue; where to live and with whom; whether or not to get married and, if so, to whom; whether or not to have children. Self-efficacy refers to our ability to make decisions like these, both large and small, and pursue our chosen courses of action.

When we lack self-confidence, we have three choices: (a) to flounder around in a state of indecision and inaction, (b) to develop self-confidence, or (c) to act according to others' judgments and expectations regardless of our own needs and desires. This last alternative is the easiest and most common course. After all, we have been taught that if we obey authority and pursue the "right" goals, we will be rewarded. However, we eventually discover a problem. If we do not feel free to direct our own lives, we feel selfless and dissatisfied.

This is not to say that we must be utterly egocentric and defiant in order to have healthy self-esteem. Not at all. We may devote our energy to doing what others want us to do; however, the desire and decision to do so must be our own. Ask yourself: am I making this choice freely, or am I feeling compelled to pursue approval and security at all costs? Am I evaluating the situation and carefully choosing my actions, or am I doing what is expected without reference to my own judgment? Do I respect my own path, or am I "putting up with it" because I feel unable to do otherwise? We will not like ourselves (or make our best possible decisions) if we are feeling *compelled* by a need for recognition and approval, or by a fear of failure.

When we suspend our ability to think, judge, and make our own choices out of fear and lack of confidence, we experience the ultimate rejection of our selves. Giving up self-determination is a sign of low self-esteem *and* an attack on self-esteem.

Why is failing to think and act independently a sign of low self-esteem? If we liked ourselves, we could afford to risk making mistakes. If we liked ourselves, we could risk being disapproved of, because our self-esteem would not depend on everyone else's approval. Thus, failing to think and act freely usually indicates chronic feelings of inadequacy, fear, and low self-esteem.

When we abandon our ability to act freely and independently, we are rejecting ourselves. It is as though our selves were jumping up and down yelling, "Okay, try this. Hey! How about doing that? . . . Why are you wasting your time with that? Listen to me!" But we just roll along and ignore our true inner voice. We pursue whatever goals we've been encouraged to pursue—like slenderness. We act in response to compelling anxieties and insecurities and hope that success will bring us approval and feelings of self-efficacy. Very often we can get the approval we were looking for, but if we ignore our inner voice, we feel selfless and ineffective anyway.

When we lack self-efficacy, we try to base our self-esteem on other sources. Dr. Branden calls this "pseudo-self-esteem." We attain pseudo-self-esteem by reaching goals we value such as academic success, professional success, and physical beauty. Pseudo-self-esteem is destined to be *low and unstable* no matter what level of popularity, accomplishment, or attractiveness we reach. Low, because we are unable to appreciate our accomplishments when they are the fruits of "forced" labor. Unstable, because the inevitable ups and downs of life keep pseudo-self-esteem on a roller coaster.

Does authentic self-esteem also suffer from the "downs" of life? Not in the same way. Failure and loss make everyone feel bad—but bad about what? People who have authentic self-esteem mourn specific failures or losses. People who have pseudo-self-esteem *blame themselves.* There is a profound difference between dissatisfaction with a particular behavior or event and dissatisfaction with yourself.

While suffering with our preoccupation, we struggle to attain diet/weight control and "attractiveness" in order to boost and maintain our pseudo-self-esteem. At the same time, we are striving for self-efficacy. Consciously or unconsciously, self-control and self-determination are major issues for us. We feel out of control. We do not know what to do when we are dissatisfied, and we feel a desperate need for more control. We begin to believe that if only this elusive "control" could be attained, greater satisfaction and fulfillment would surely follow.

This yearning for control is actually a yearning for self-determination. It is our selves saying, "I want to choose, but instead I'm struggling for approval and acceptance. I don't like living this way, but I'm terrified that people will reject me." In order to feel good about ourselves, we search for ways to take more control over ourselves and our lives. And from all sources we are instructed: "Improve your life and get control of yourself: restrict your diet and lose weight." We become quite excited by this solution. We hope that we can finally "control ourselves" and "improve ourselves" by jumping on the weight-loss wagon.

Almost immediately we run into a distressing problem: we find that seemingly irrational desires and needs from within us attempt to undermine our newfound control. We know that we want to lose weight. We know that we want to restrict our diets. Thus, for the first time in a long time, we know exactly what we want to do. When our need for food overrides our determination to lose weight, we feel that yet another force is challenging and eroding our attempts to act on the basis of our own judgment. Furthermore, we assume that we have only ourselves to blame. *We want to base our food choices on our new decision to eat less and lose weight—which makes us feel a little more powerful and in control. But this task turns into a terrible struggle between our goals and our bodies' very real demands.*

Here is a way for dissatisfied approval seekers to fight their feelings of inefficacy and inadequacy without questioning societal, parental, peer, or self-expectations. We can accept everything that is enslaving us (for more on this, see Chapter 6) and proceed to *fight for rational independence* from our bodies' tyrannical demands for "too much" food. In this way we can continue to take little personal initiative in areas of our lives that matter, and not work toward authentic, positive self-esteem, yet feel as though we are struggling for personal progress.

Think of all the satisfaction and feelings of self-control we can derive from resisting "bad" desires to eat many times a day. If we look at our lives as a series of options, judgments, decisions, and actions, we can see that when we control our eating we inject our lives with independent judgments, decisions, and actions. The sole focus is on diet, perhaps exercise, and weight, but at least we are taking action—fighting for greater control and greater satisfaction—rather than just sitting on our feelings of inadequacy and dissatisfaction.

My workshop participants describe feelings of inefficacy and low self-esteem despite their successful and independent facades. *Dietary and weight control has become equated with control of themselves and their lives.* If they maintain diet/weight control, they feel as though their self-efficacy and self-esteem are intact; otherwise, they feel out of control.

My workshop members also explore their beliefs and expectations about "what it would be like to be model thin." Becky had a vivid image that speaks for many people who are preoccupied with diet and weight. Becky said that she would experience the world as a "brighter, happier place": all her decisions would be easier to make; socializing would be easier and more satisfying; men would flock around her; buying clothes would be enjoyable instead of painful. . . . In short, she said that everything would be better because the "dark, heavy cloud" of dislike for her body and desperation about eating would be gone.

These unrealistic expectations of the "thin life" are understandable if we recognize what Becky expected to gain from diet/weight control: stable, positive self-esteem based on newly attained self-efficacy. *If* weight loss could have provided this, her expectations for an incomparably better life wouldn't have been so unrealistic. Low self-esteem and a lack of self-efficacy *do* hang over people like dark clouds. Low self-esteem makes it impossible to feel satisfied with one's performance, causes endless doubts regarding one's individuality, independence, and lovability, and makes new situations—social or otherwise—unpleasant and difficult. Becky also hoped that losing weight would end her painful preoccupation with diet and weight. Diet/weight preoccupation also hangs over people like a dark cloud; however, weight loss almost never frees people from it. Since weight loss is not a magic cure for low self-esteem or diet/weight preoccupation, Becky's image of the thin life was totally unrealistic.

Irrational expectations of the thin life are very harmful. If you expect your entire life to be transformed into a blissful state, it's not surprising that you pursue slenderness regardless of cost! However, deep down inside, you know that your expectations are unrealistic. That knowledge can actually make you fear and avoid weight loss.[2] What if you attain your goal weight and life is no better? What if you don't automatically become Superwoman? What if you still don't feel lovable? What if you still have trouble in social situations? Better to dream, we might think, rather than struggle to our dream only to have it crushed.

Most of you will find that your desperation for weight loss and dietary control reflects a desperation for strength, self-improvement, love, and happiness. You want to feel good about yourself and your life—that is natural and right. You deserve the greatest possible fulfillment. The question is, will dietary control and weight loss truly lead you to that goal?

REPLACING PERFECTIONISM AND NEGATIVISM

Are you a perfectionist? If so, then you need to know that perfectionism goes hand in hand with disliking ourselves and seeing things in a negative light. All three promote dissatisfaction and despair.

As perfectionists, we ensure that we will never be satisfied with ourselves or our accomplishments. We have prejudged ourselves as "no good," and by being perfectionists we rationalize that judgment. Our search for perfection may sound like a positive thing—like a search for greatness. In truth, *a search for perfection is always a search for fault*. In our quest for perfection, we must search for fault no matter how much merit we find, because perfection exists only where fault does not. Perfection is not an abundance of merit but a lack of fault. If an abundance of merit gets in our way, we can simply intensify our scrutiny and extend our search for fault.

Imagine that a leader from another planet sent two women to earth with two different tasks. One was told to seek perfection, so that upon her return she could point to all that was perfect. The other was told to seek goodness, so that upon her return she could point to all that was good. What would each of the women report? The former would probably report that her search was fruitless because the world was an evil and horrible place. The latter would probably report that she hardly knew where to begin, because there was so much good in the world. Which emissary would return depressed and dissatisfied, she who sought perfection, or she who sought goodness? If you had to be one of these women, which one would you want to be?

Perfectionism does not serve any purpose well, and it promotes misery and dissatisfaction. If you can see and believe that being a perfectionist necessarily harms rather than helps you, then you can let go of it. None of us wants to be unhappy. We cling to perfectionism and negativism because they seem to help us survive. As you read the following list of "benefits," ask: "Am I looking for that? Is there a more effective way to meet my needs?"

Six "Benefits" of Perfectionism

1. Perfectionism offers a rationalization and justification for our irrational self-hatred and disapproval. If perfection is our goal, then as long as imperfection can be found, we (and our achievements) are not "good enough," and our dissatisfaction seems justified.

2. Perfectionism offers a desperately needed vision of fulfillment. "I would have been satisfied with that term paper

if only . . ." "I would like my body if only . . ." "I could be happy if only . . ." "I would like myself if only. . . ." We fool ourselves into thinking that if only we could do or be better, we would be happy. We cling to this vision to get through each day.

3. Perfectionism offers to keep our true hopes and expectations low so that we cannot be let down. "I'm not going to expect to succeed because I don't want to be disappointed—I'd rather expect the worst and be pleasantly surprised." Sound familiar? Perfectionists can employ this rationale to an extreme. Failure is assured as long as goals are completely unrealistic; thus, any *unexpected* failure is avoided.

4. Perfectionism offers to protect us from the fear that we can't "stay this good." When we do something well, we sometimes wonder, "What can I do for an encore? What if I never do anything as impressive again? What if it's all downhill from here?" If nothing we do is ever "good enough," then we may avoid the fear that we cannot live up to past performances.

5. Perfectionism offers delusions of omnipotence. We envision a "perfect" self because it makes us feel at least potentially respectable and lovable. We think that we must be perfect—and thereby better than everyone else—in order to earn self-love and others' love.

6. Perfectionism offers us a reason to forgive ourselves. Deep down we know that it is impossible to be perfect, so we are not to blame for falling short. We give ourselves conditional forgiveness,

which is not liberating. As long as we are perfectionists, we can feel guilty and upset without taking responsibility—without using our power to end our dissatisfaction and feelings of inadequacy.

These are a few of the ways in which we can use perfectionism to maintain enough self-respect for survival. Perfectionism is difficult to give up because we are afraid of losing our ability to cope. The worse we feel, the more we cling to our methods of coping. Furthermore, perfectionism is addictive. We get something from it, we have become accustomed to it, and we are therefore afraid to give it up.

If you are a perfectionist, you can choose to stop being one. I am not suggesting that you stop doing your best, nor am I suggesting that you refuse to see and react to your mistakes. I am suggesting that you look for the good in yourself and your world instead of looking for perfection (and thereby, fault).

Any true benefits you sought with perfectionism can be attained more easily in other ways. You can set ambitious goals, and work toward them as diligently as you like, without being a perfectionist. A perfectionist sets unattainable goals. Wouldn't you *like* to have goals that can be happily realized?

What if you do not realize a goal after letting go of perfectionism? Then you can discover that an unrealized goal is your own creation, which you can continue to pursue or change in any way you like. While your goal is an absolute—perfection—you have no control over it, and it haunts you. Once you create your own goals they can be wonderful confidence builders instead of specters of failure.

When we give up perfectionism, we also

give up certain positive feelings. We stop picturing ourselves as perfect and omnipotent. At first this may feel like a decrease in self-esteem, but it is not. Giving up any kind of addiction feels bad at first but soon thereafter improves our lives. Many of us have been taught to think that we have to be shockingly extraordinary—better than everyone else—in order to be special and worthwhile. Once we unlearn that absurd lesson, we no longer need to be perfect or "better than" others to feel good about ourselves. Our self-esteem improves, and our lives become much more satisfying.

One of the most painful parts of being a perfectionist is that we tend to be very unforgiving of our own and others' faults. We have been taught that forgiveness requires one of two things: justification or penance. In truth, forgiveness requires only respect and love. We can choose to forgive if we want to. We are always free to choose.

When I was in high school, I wrote a paper on the internment of Japanese people in the United States during World War II. I was interested in this subject because my grandfather was kept in U.S. concentration camps throughout the war. As part of my research, I asked my grandfather to tell me about his experiences. While I waited for his reply, I read about it in textbooks, and the more I read, the angrier I became.

When I read my grandfather's account of his abduction and internment, I was amazed and frustrated. Not just because of his horrible experiences, but because of the way he described those experiences. Every paragraph revealed his nonjudgmental and forgiving viewpoint. He did not just describe the bad conditions or the ways in which he was persecuted. He described those who had treated him well, and those he was able to help. Now I see the wisdom behind his viewpoint.

In order to live peacefully and happily in the world, we cannot blame ourselves or others for mistakes. We must hold on to the knowledge that each of us acts wrongly only when we are afraid, desperate, or needy. Forgiveness is one of the keys to happiness.[3] In order to like ourselves, others, and our world, we need to forgive all transgressions, real or imagined. It doesn't matter what we have done, nor what anyone else has done to us. We cannot be happy unless we live in a loving way, and a central part of loving is forgiving.

Better yet, we can *avoid judgmental attitudes and behavior* in the first place. Suppose that you see a man being abusive to a woman. You might think, "What a jerk! I'd like to see him get a taste of his own medicine!" On the other hand, you could think, "That poor man. He must be hurting to act like that." The first reaction is highly judgmental and unforgiving; the second reaction is empathetic. The first reaction looks to inflict punishment (which usually leads to more abusive behavior); the second reaction looks to understand and, perhaps, help. The first reaction is based on *our* pain; the second reaction is based on the understanding that, deep inside, we all want to be good to ourselves and others, but our true selves can get lost beneath pain and fear.

Many of us are in the habit of standing in judgment over everyone and everything. However, once we focus on understanding instead of judging, it becomes the most natural way to live. Our capacity to be understanding and forgiving then grows automatically because our lives become better. Once we relax and let our true selves take charge, we automatically develop and repeat what feels best.

When I read a beautiful book called *Love is Letting Go of Fear* (by Dr. Gerald Jampolsky), I realized how much *my efforts to become less judgmental had boosted my self-esteem.* Dr. Jampolsky provided a concrete explanation of what I had already experienced: that when I judge others, I also judge myself; that if I do not forgive others, I cannot forgive myself. I tried to be less judgmental for other people's sakes. As a result, I have learned to understand and forgive myself as well.

This is not to say that I never make harsh judgments. Sometimes I do. But now that I see how harmful it is, I find it much easier to forgive. In forgiving, I set myself free to love and appreciate, which are the true sources of self-acceptance and fulfillment.

If you tend to isolate yourself, or if you feel close to very few people, then the most effective way to strengthen your self-esteem is to *reach out.* You need and deserve to be loved by others. You need and deserve to experience the joy of loving and trusting others. If you could accomplish this thing only—to infuse your life with love on every level—you could not continue to dislike yourself, or be a perfectionist, or see things in a negative light. This is because by loving others you reveal and fully enjoy the best of yourself, other people, and everything around you.

How can you infuse your life with love? Certainly not by waiting to fall in love, nor by waiting for others to love you. Certainly not by pretending to be the person you think everyone else wants you to be. You will have to reach out, open up, learn to listen, talk, and cry. You will have to find the courage to show that you want to know and appreciate others in a deep and profound way. You will have to allow others to know and appreciate you in the same way. You will have to look for goodness instead of looking for fault, and you will have to learn to communicate your feelings even when it's scary and risky. As you do these things, you will find it much easier to give yourself the same understanding and love.

Many people maintain that unless you love yourself, you cannot love others. I'm not sure whether that is true or not. But it is undoubtedly true that the more fully you love and accept yourself, the more fully you can love and accept others *and vice versa:* the more fully you love and accept others, the more fully you can love and accept yourself.

APPRECIATING OUR IMPERFECT AND LOVABLE SELVES

You can stop judging yourself against unrealistic and irrational standards. You can train yourself to think: "My body is wonderful and beautiful as it is. I can be proud of myself even if my achievements are not perfect. I am completely lovable even though some people do not like me. I do the best I can, and that is always good enough. My mistakes can teach and help me. I am a good person, and in my own way I make the world a nicer place."

Try this exercise. Every morning when you wake up, talk to yourself for a minute or so. Remind yourself—*aloud*—that you're not perfect, but you're perfectly fine. Then say to yourself: "I'm glad to be me. I'm a valuable, loving person. Not only that, it's a beautiful day and I'm psyched!" (Put it in your own words.)

When you go to bed at night, take a minute to think about what you did and how you felt about it. First, appreciate yourself for all that went well during the day. If you regret something, make peace with yourself about it. Acknowledge it, think about what you learned, how you might be able to rectify the mistake, and what you need in order to avoid the same mistake again. Then give yourself a break: it's okay to make mistakes. You're still a good person. Congratulate yourself on another day well lived.

The things you say to yourself have a big effect on how you think and feel. Most of us have learned to be very critical of ourselves. It is as though we had tapes playing in our heads with someone saying: "You're such a jerk." "That's not good enough." "You're so stupid." "You're so clumsy." "Well, it could have been worse, but. . . ." The messages on these tapes are unhelpful and undeserved. Worse yet, they reinforce feelings of inadequacy.

In order to feel better about yourself, you have to replace these critical tapes with something positive. For instance, instead of thinking, "That's not good enough," you can think, "This is very good, but let's see if I can make it even better." Instead of thinking, "You're so clumsy," you can think, "Whoops—I didn't see that in my way." In addition, *try to practice a positive outlook on yourself and your life.*

Read over the "Happy and Healthy Thoughts" that follow. These are the kinds of thoughts that need to become an integral part of you. Make a copy of the list, and put it somewhere so that you can read it at least once a day without going out of your way. For instance, on the wall across from the toilet is a nice unavoidable spot. Or carry the copy around with you and read it when standing in lines, on the john, or in the bathtub.

I give the above "assignment" to all of my workshop participants. Over time I have found that some people do it without difficulty, while others have a very hard time. In general, the harder it is, the more the person needs to read it. If you find yourself resisting and forgetting a lot, don't think that it's because it's a silly exercise. Chances are that you *really* need to do it. Otherwise, it wouldn't be so hard to do.

Improving your self-esteem will probably be a long, hard task. At times you may feel like you're just going through the motions of self-appreciation; you may feel that you're "faking" positive self-esteem. That's okay! Just keep practicing and faking it. If you persevere, you'll begin to feel it as well.

I used to be a self-destructive perfectionist. I was an excellent student, but I never felt that I was working hard enough, or that my achievements were legitimate and meaningful. If you think that academic or professional *achievement* is going to make you feel good about yourself, think again. Achievement alone won't do it for you no matter how much you achieve. Achievement will not silence that irrational voice that says: "You think you're pretty good, don't you? Ha! Think again. You're an egotistical idiot whose accomplishments are worthless. People are going to find that out any day now."

Learning to Love Ourselves

HAPPY AND HEALTHY THOUGHTS*

Read these statements every day until they become part of your thinking. Do not memorize them.

1. I am a unique and precious human being, always doing the best I can, always growing in wisdom and love.

2. I don't need to prove myself to anyone—not even to myself—for I know that I am perfectly fine as I am.

3. I make my own decisions and assume responsibility for any mistakes. However, I refuse to feel shame or guilt about them. I do the best I can, and that is 100 percent good enough.

4. I am not my actions. I am the actor. My actions may be good or bad. That doesn't make me good or bad.

5. Whenever I am tempted to punish myself, I remember to be kind and gentle instead. I know that in order to be the best I can be, I need forgiveness and understanding.

6. I know that it is okay to need. I try to keep in touch with my needs so that I can respond to them.

7. I know that others cannot be expected to read my mind or to guess my needs. In fairness to them and to me, I ask for what I need.

8. I deserve to be appreciated. When others show their appreciation, I embrace it with open arms. I never try to deny or diminish my value.

9. I live one day at a time and do first things first.

10. I take great pride in what I do, in what I value, and in the way I live, for I truly believe in myself.

11. My mistakes and nonsuccess do not make me a louse, a failure, or whatever. They only prove that I am imperfect, that is, human. It's wonderful to be human.

12. I love myself, absolutely and unconditionally, for that is what I truly need and deserve.

* Adapted from "Happy Homework," author unknown.

Don't believe that voice. It is utterly wrong. Respond with something more accurate. Perhaps something like: "I am a wonderful, beautiful person exactly as I am. I will face my desire for perfection, let it pass over me and through me, and then let it go. Where a perfectionist was, only I will remain: imperfect and fine, ever loving and ever lovable."[4]

Questions to Ask Your Judgmental Voice

Every road to self-acceptance and positive self-esteem is long and rocky. You will probably find yourself battling irrational self-hatred and guilt. The following questions can help you bow out of those battles and thereby win.

Question #1: Would I Ever Judge a Friend As Harshly As I Am Judging Myself?

If a dear friend of mine acted as I did (or felt as I did, or gained weight) would I think that she was a bad person? We are our own most critical judges. In fact, most of us are much harder on ourselves than on those we love. The primary reason for this is clear: we don't love ourselves. Since it is impossible to magically develop self-love, we must work toward it step by step. Act as though you respect and appreciate yourself until it becomes true. *Always try to give yourself the loving support, praise, forgiveness, and tolerance that you grant your best-loved friends and family.* Know that this is appropriate: you deserve to be treated well. Know that this is right: it is moral to love and be good to yourself.

Question #2: What Could I Have Done Differently?

If you feel bad about something, be sure that your regret is within reason. We often blame ourselves and feel guilty even though we've acted in *the best way open to us.*

Why would we be so irrational? There are many possible reasons. Some of us automatically respond to negative events with guilt. When someone treats us poorly, we feel guilty. When someone makes us angry, we feel guilty for responding with anger. If we hurt someone by mistake, we feel guilty. If we decide to end a painful relationship, we feel guilty. I use guilt as an example because a few years ago I realized that my "favorite" feeling—the feeling I chose most often—was guilt. Through some convoluted logic, I thought that feeling guilty "made up for" being a worthless person. I was caught in two misconceptions: that I was worthless, and that guilt was an effective form of atonement.

Another reason why some of us condemn ourselves in irrational ways is that we carry around unreasonable "authorities" inside our heads—authorities we don't even agree with. For instance, suppose you were taught that expressing anger is unacceptable no matter what the circumstances. You may have rejected that value on a conscious level yet continue to feel very bad about expressing anger.

The simple question "What could I have done differently?" can help you avoid the trap of irrational self-condemnation. Sometimes you *can* pinpoint some better way in which you might have behaved. Then you can learn something, or get what you need to do it differently next time, and feel good about *that*. If it is possible to "undo" your mistake (by apologizing or whatever), then do so. In any case, self-recrimination and guilt are unproductive for you and everyone else involved. Try some other options.

Question #3: Did I Do the Best I Could? Am I Doing the Best I Can?

We often look back on our behavior *with new insights* and think, "Good grief! How could I have done that? I could have done better." But it is hardly fair to judge harshly on the basis of new insights and perspective. That is like looking back on a flunked arithmetic test in adulthood and thinking, "How could I not have known how to add and subtract when it's so easy!"

Even in the present we sometimes think, "What's wrong with me? I can do better than this!" Try to skip over that thought and move straight to: "This isn't exactly what I want to be doing; I think I'll try something else instead." Beware of assuming that you are not really trying if you are not getting the results you want.

We all tend to act like frustrated athletes. Over and over I have watched players become angry with themselves: "What are you doing? Concentrate—you're not concentrating!" We try so hard, yet we don't seem to believe that we're doing the best we can. "But I've seen myself do better!" we cry. "I really can do better than this." We miss the fact that our superior performance was achieved at a different time, when we were in a different state of mind and set of circumstances. If we can recreate that state of mind and set of circumstances, we can probably match our past performance. But if we

do not manage to do that, then we must accept and appreciate our current "best," whatever that may be.

In every moment we need to remember that "that was then and this is now," and then choose to *live in the present.* Self-acceptance can only be experienced in the present. If we do not accept and appreciate ourselves now, we may do it later, but even then we will be accepting and appreciating ourselves in the (new) present. Over and over people tell me that they'll feel better about themselves when they are thinner, or when they are more independent, or "tomorrow." The only time you can truly choose self-acceptance is in the present. You do not know what the future will bring except new moments—when you will again have to choose whether or not to appreciate yourself.

You can choose unconditional self-acceptance instead of all the measuring, comparing, and judging you have been taught to do. At every moment, you have the choice of self-acceptance and appreciation, whether you are at your best or at your worst.

FILLING OUR LIVES WITH LOVE

Everyone wants to be appreciated and loved. We have to face up to the fact that we cannot be loved by everyone precisely in the way we want; however, we can choose a way of life that is loving, and thereby ensure that we will experience and share love. When we are loving and being loved well, we can feel at home in the world.

Have you ever noticed that the world often acts like a mirror? Whatever you send out returns.[5] Have you ever noticed that simply giving makes you feel good? Dr. Jampolsky puts it another way: "All that I give is given to myself."[6] Experiment with the following exercises:

1. Smile and say hello to toll booth operators, cashiers, waitresses, secretaries, gas station attendants, and other service people. Take five or ten seconds to focus your attention and goodwill on someone. Wish her a good day; give thanks in a sincere way. She'll usually appreciate it and return your smile and goodwill. (Don't worry when it doesn't work. That person's suffering was too great for you to break through.)

2. Look for and focus on people's strengths. Ask yourself: "What do I like about this person?" instead of "What do I think of this person?" If you begin to measure yourself against someone—comparing and competing in your own mind—replace that line of thought with "What can I learn from this person?" Our competitive world has taught us that other people's strengths highlight our weaknesses. We needn't accept that unhelpful lesson. We can be enriched by others' strengths instead of competing with them.

3. Express your appreciation for others. Insincere flattery is ugly and offensive; however, sincere appreciation helps other people feel good about themselves and good about you. Also, when you make someone else feel good, it tends to make you feel good.

4. Think of ways in which you can make a difference in the lives of people around you. Don't choose anything difficult or painful—that isn't necessary or helpful. Just find something nice that you can do.

LETTING GO OF FEAR

Do you ever get the feeling that if someone says "no" to your request, or if someone disapproves of you, or if you fail at something, then the world will crash in around you? I spent much of my life burdened with that feeling, and it had a crippling effect. Unless I was sure of success, I was afraid to act or make requests. My fear robbed me of personal freedom.

If you could accept and love yourself unconditionally, then you would not feel so vulnerable; however, since that love doesn't reappear overnight, you need to find immediate ways to work through fear and anxiety. Try thinking through the most painful results that could possibly ensue from the rejection or failure. Ask yourself, "Would it really be so unbearable?" If it doesn't seem unbearable, go for it! If the results are actually painful, you can learn another valuable lesson: you can handle challenges well and life goes on.

Keep these ideas in mind:

You Can Handle "No"

When someone says "no" to you, you are still as worthy, capable, and valuable as you were before. In fact, most "no's" do not carry serious consequences. I learned this in a funny way. I became a salesperson. I didn't sell in a store, where people are expecting and wanting to see salespeople. I sold expensive pots and pans door-to-door, where people hate to see salespeople.

At first it was incredibly hard to hear "no," even if it was said politely. I hated *asking* people to sign away their hard-earned money, knowing that they might very well refuse. But the more I heard both "yes" and "no," the more I realized that "no" was just an inevitable part of the process, and that I could accept it comfortably.

This is true in all kinds of situations: "no" is just part of the process, and can be accepted comfortably. If you never ask questions, then you can avoid a lot of "no's", but you'll automatically avoid a lot of "yesses" too.

Think about job hunting, for example. If you never ask anyone for a job, you'll never be turned down, but you probably won't find a job, either. Think about making friends. If you never ask anyone out, you'll never be turned down, but you'll only be able to make friends with people who ask you. "Nothing ventured, nothing gained."

The best way to get what you want and need from others is to ask for it. A friend of mine, Julie, asked Samantha how she managed to make so many friends. Samantha could have said that it was because she was very warm and understanding or because she was a good listener, all of which was true. But she said, "I ask everyone I like to come over or do something with me. Sometimes we become friends."

This story contains a helpful lesson. We can learn that rejection and failure needn't destroy us, and thereby free ourselves to try. Most of us are afraid to ask for anything, whether it is a job, a date, a favor, or some needed assistance. We feel vulnerable be-

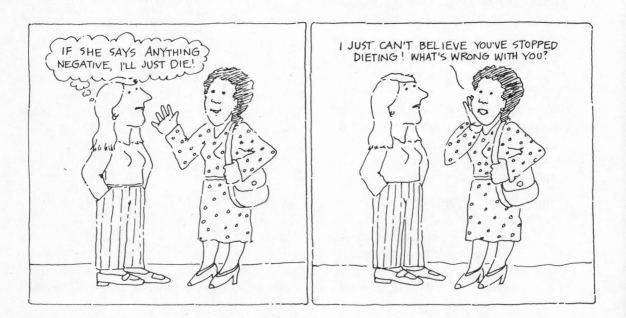

cause we are afraid of rejection. Learn to ask for what you want. People cannot be expected to read your mind. You will be the same, wonderful, lovable, deserving person no matter how many times you hear "no." And, the more you let yourself hear "no," the less scary it will be, and the more you will hear "yes."

Disapproval Won't Kill You!

When someone disapproves of your actions, you can either agree and learn from the mistake *or* disagree and accept the fact that different people have different values. Either way you are no less worthy or less valuable than you were before. No one can avoid disapproval—it's another fact of life like the word "no." But you can learn to take it in stride by remembering that you are valuable, respectable, and lovable no matter who disapproves.

Failure Neither Dooms nor Defines You

When you fail at a particular task, *you* are not a failure: you are the same able, wonderful person you were before who, like everyone else, isn't perfect. I'll bet that you thought failure was a sin, a disaster, an unbearable embarrassment, a sign of stupidity, or proof of your "inadequacy"! It's none of those things. Failure is just another inevitable part of life. It shows that you are a fallible human being who is willing to take on challenges.

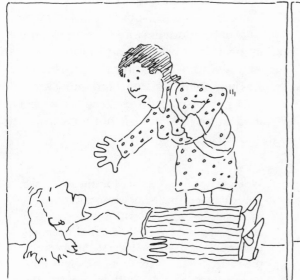 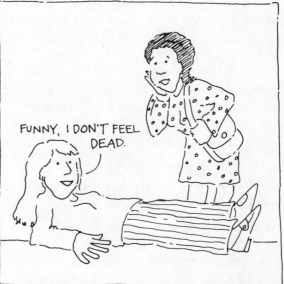

You Are Fine No Matter How Long It Takes to Progress

As you take on the tasks and goals in this book, you will make some mistakes and enjoy many victories. If you are not progressing toward freedom as you would like to, you are still a fine and capable person—you are not "bad." Push yourself forward, but don't ever punish yourself.

In my workshops I always encourage participants to stop talking about weight and eating behavior in moralistic terms ("bad food," "good food," "bad eating," "I was bad"). Whenever someone says, "I was bad yesterday. I binged like you wouldn't believe," I say something like "Did your binge transform you from the wonderful person you are into a bad person?" At first, many members respond by shifting their judgmental attitudes to different standards. Consequently, I often hear something like this: "I was really bad yesterday. I got so anxious that I started dieting again." After a while, however, most members begin to speak *and think* about their eating as choices without moral implications.

Remember: *you* are not "bad." You sometimes make choices that cause you pain—but that doesn't make you any "less good" than you were before.

CHOOSING PEACE OVER PUNISHMENT

As you work toward freedom from the diet/weight obsession, try to observe and notice your progress *without judging or blaming*. What do I mean by that? Let's suppose that I find myself weight-loss dieting after a year of attempting to eat spontaneously. My first reaction might be "What's *wrong* with me? Why can't I just stop torturing myself? I will not diet anymore if it kills me." Later that day let's suppose I find myself looking for bulges of fat at my waist. My first reaction might be "This is really bad. I shouldn't be doing this. I'll never let go of my preoccupation this way."

What's the problem? The problem is that my reactions are couched in blame. I am chastising myself instead of accepting myself. I am seeing my actions as my "bad behavior" instead of as my "present behavior." If I acknowledge that I have begun to diet and scrutinize my body *without judging that behavior or myself* as "bad," then I leave myself free to respond to that information without guilt, discouragement, or depression. I can see what I am doing, deal with my actions without judgments of "good" or "bad," and then choose my subsequent action based on what I really want.

There is a relaxed, spontaneous, noncompulsive eater hidden away inside each of us. Our job is to observe and help ourselves emerge without hindering the process with value judgments, blame, and punishment. This is not easy to do because we've been trained to be judgmental, but we can learn and practice new patterns.

When we plant a rose seed in the earth, we notice that it is small, but we do not criticize it as "rootless and stemless." We treat it as a seed, giving it the water and nourishment required of a seed. When it first shoots up out of the earth, we don't condemn it as immature and underdeveloped; nor do we criticize the buds for not being open when they appear. We stand in wonder at the process taking place and give the plant the care it needs at each stage of its development. The rose is a rose from the time it is a seed to the time it dies. Within it, at all times, it contains its whole potential . . . at each state, at each moment, it is perfectly all right as it is.[7]

You, too, are perfectly all right as you are at every stage of development. That is not to say that none of your behavior is self-destructive—some of it is. But by giving yourself the encouragement, respect, and love that you need (in place of the criticism, blame, and rejection that you don't need), you can progress much more easily and happily.

PERSONAL QUESTIONS: BEFRIENDING YOURSELF

1. During your childhood and adolescence, how did the significant people in your life (such as parents and peers) treat you? How did they appreciate you? How did they criticize you?

2. How do you criticize yourself (currently)?

3. How do you appreciate yourself? For instance, do you praise yourself mentally? Do you often think, "That was well done" or "I'm a loving person"? Why or why not?

4. Which do you focus on more, your strengths or your weaknesses? Why? Is your focus helpful?

5. Write down three negative statements that you repeatedly say to yourself. For each of these statements, write down one or more positive statements that you can use as replacements.

6. Are you a perfectionist? If so, how is your perfectionism helpful? How does your perfectionism hurt you?

7. Think back over the major decisions you have made. Who or what influenced you most?

8. Do you think that any of your decisions were, in a sense, made for you? If so, how do you feel about that?

9. How much does *anxiety* influence your behavior, life-style, and decisions? How do you feel about it? What would you like to change?

10. Do you have confidence in your own judgment? Why or why not?

11. Do you feel that you are directing your life? Why or why not? If not, who or what is directing your life? How can you consciously take responsibility for more of your decisions and goals?

12. In what ways are you a loving and supportive person?

13.   Do you want to become a more loving person? If so, how can you begin?

14.   Do you like yourself? Are you proud of the person you have (so far) become? Why or why not? Is your self-evaluation predominantly rational or irrational?

15.   What qualities do you respect in people, and what qualities do you dislike? Make two lists.

POSITIVE QUALITIES	NEGATIVE QUALITIES

16.   Look over your list and star your strengths. Make a separate list of all the items you starred. Add your personal skills and accomplishments.

MY STRENGTHS, SKILLS, AND ACCOMPLISHMENTS

17.   Make a separate list of characteristics you would like to develop or change, and actions that might lead to each of these goals.

CHARACTERISTICS	PLANS OF ACTION

18. Select the most important goal listed above, and answer the following questions:

• Why do you want to work toward this particular goal? How will it help you? Will the pursuit and/or achievement of this goal make you happier?

• What resources do you have to help you achieve your goal?

• What will your challenges be?

• What steps must you take to reach your goal?

19. Make a list of all the benefits and the costs of loving and respecting yourself unconditionally.

LOVING AND RESPECTING MYSELF UNCONDITIONALLY	
BENEFITS	COSTS

20. Do you value unconditional self-respect and acceptance? In other words, do you think that unconditionally accepting, respecting, and loving yourself would benefit you and those you love? Why or why not?

21.   Imagine for a moment that you are someone else—an imaginary close friend who loves you completely and unconditionally. Write a letter that explains all the reasons behind your feelings. (Why does this person love you so much? Why did she/he choose you for a friend?)

Dear _____ : (Fill in your real name.)

Do you know how much I love you? I think you do. But do you know why I love you so dearly? Let me tell you. The first time I met you, I knew that I wanted to be your friend because _____
_____ ,
_____ . I love you because _____
and I love you because _____ .
Just being with you _____ .
You don't have to _____ because
_____ .

I admire you in so many ways. Here's an incomplete list. I admire:

a. _____ .
b. _____ .
c. _____ .
d. _____ .
e. _____ .
f. _____ .
g. _____ .

Every now and then you act as though _____ ,
but it's okay because actually, _____ .
(Continue the letter as you like.)

I would be afraid to write a letter like this to most people, but I wasn't afraid to be completely open with you because _____
_____ .

                                    Your loving friend,

P.S.

22.   How did it make you feel to write that letter? Why?

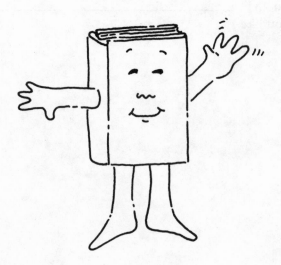

6
SORTING OUT
OUR VALUES

Imagine that you have just walked, all alone, into an unknown city surrounded by walls that stretch upward as far as you can see. Within this city you talk to people, but everyone treats you poorly and eventually makes one or both of the following statements: "Outsiders are hated and feared if they speak to cityfolk" and "Those who do not speak are fools only fit to be slaves." You soon find that the situation is hopeless. If you talk to people, they hate and fear you; if you don't talk, they try to enslave you. Not wanting to knock your head against a wall any longer, you try to leave. But suppose you cannot find the gate, or the gate is locked. Suppose you are forced to remain in this society indefinitely. How would you feel? How would you act?

Anyone in this nightmare would hope to awaken as quickly as possible. But if it were not a nightmare—if it were real—the situation would cause feelings of frustration, *helplessness*, and (eventually) *inadequacy*. Even an unusually capable, well-adjusted,

and self-assured person would eventually feel helpless and inadequate in that situation.

Chronic feelings of inadequacy, helplessness, and a tremendous desire for control are shared by most of us. I am constantly hearing "I just want to be in control." What are we seeking to control? What are we really searching for? Underneath our desire for control of diet and weight, we are longing for control of ourselves and our lives. We want to ensure that people will love, respect, appreciate, and hear us. In short, we are longing for satisfaction and fulfillment. Why, as we struggle toward that universal goal, do we feel inadequate and out of control?

Most of us are forever trying to respond to contradictory and/or destructive beliefs and expectations. We are like the captive stranger, in a sense, except that most of us are unaware of the no-win situations we face.

For instance, at a young age we learn that

achievement is valuable and good, and that we should perform to the best of our abilities. However, most girls also learn that we should not threaten and alienate the opposite sex by "outdoing them" in things they value.

What things do they value? Let's look at a few examples. In childhood, boys highly value athletic ability, and they are taught that it is a great disgrace to be beaten by a girl. By junior high school, sports have been segregated by gender, and academic achievement is starting to be an issue. In adulthood, careers become the major issue, and most men have been taught that they should make more money and have a higher-status job than their girlfriends or wives.

Evidence indicates that most girls and women cooperate in keeping male peers on top. Studies show that until early adolescence, girls perform as well as or better than boys in every subject. However, beginning in junior high school, girls' aspiration, motivation, and performance decline.[1] Numerous studies have shown that from that time on, many women are motivated to avoid excellence in school, particularly if they accept and eventually want to fulfill women's traditional role of wife and mother.[2]

Of course, the opposite lesson has also been learned: that it is important to achieve, succeed, and thereby gain satisfaction and status. Thus women are faced with a no-win situation, particularly if very talented. Either we perform below our abilities and feel bad about our relatively poor performance, or we fulfill our potential and suffer the resulting social rejection.

Most girls and women do one of three things: (a) avoid competing with less gifted males, (b) purposely perform below potential, or (c) try to hide threatening abilities and accomplishments.

As a young tomboy, I naively chose none of the above options. Instead, I beat the boys at everything I could. Being a very athletic child, I beat them at a lot, from pull-up contests to running races. I was quite pleased with myself. But later, in dancing school with all the same boys, I wondered why no one wanted to dance with me.

Later, when academic achievement became the issue, I was no longer so naive. I chose the third alternative, and hid my test scores and report cards from male peers. I avoided coed discussions of grades. Boys started to like me and ask me out.

By the time I reached college, I had perfected this "solution" to such a degree that it was completely automatic. I wasn't even aware of hiding my academic ability and achievement. Nonetheless, my closest male friend thought that he was a smarter, better student for three and a half years. I'll never forget his shocked expression upon learning that I was to graduate ninth in our class, well ahead of him. It wasn't until much later that I realized I had not only allowed but encouraged him to believe that he was intellectually superior.

As we get older and join the work force and/or start a family, conflicting expectations and demands do not decrease; if anything, they get tougher. Most of us learn that it is important to fulfill the traditional role of wife and mother. But we cannot help but be aware that our society devalues this pursuit.

It is seen as the absence of a career, rather than a career in its own right. We soon find ourselves feeling embarrassed and inferior when people ask "What do you do?" unless we can reply with something other than "I'm just a housewife."

In our society status is determined, for the most part, by income. The more money you make, the higher your status. Women are not exempt from this hierarchy. Therefore, we face a real problem. Are we going to be "good wives and mothers" and accept low status? Or are we going to choose a traditionally feminine career and achieve slightly higher status? Or are we going to compete for a more lucrative, high-status job and be considered threatening and "masculine"? And if we are going to try for both a high-status career and motherhood, how are we going to succeed in competition with men, most of whom are themselves taken care of by their wives, and none of whom have to battle against sexism?

For the most part, our culture pretends that every woman can be a "supermom," with a good job and a beautiful, well-looked-after family. Commercials, for instance, show the relaxed, smiling housewife/professional standing by her husband as he lovingly describes her success: "My wife's incredible. She feeds the kids, she cooks the meals, she cleans the house, she goes to the office . . . and look at her, she's still beautiful." Is it surprising that we feel overwhelmed? Or is it virtually unavoidable that given the circumstances we feel inadequate, pulled apart by conflicting demands, and "out of control"?

Women are also faced with an inconsistent and irrational set of rules for behavior and personality. On the one hand, our society highly values traditionally "masculine" characteristics. Particularly in the workplace, people are rewarded for being assertive, confident, competent, levelheaded in crisis, aggressive, unemotional, and objective. But in order to be considered "feminine," one is expected to act very differently. Even mental health clinicians have characterized "healthy women" as being "more submissive, less aggressive, less adventurous, more easily influenced, less competent, more excitable in minor crises, feelings more easily hurt, more emotional and less objective"[3]— characteristics that are devalued by our society.

Once again, we find ourselves in a no-win situation. Shall we take on the expected, but devalued, feminine characteristics? Or shall we take on the more valued masculine characteristics and be stigmatized as "masculine" women?

I have had a rare and fascinating look at the way women are received if they choose the latter course. As the fiancée of a Harvard Business School (HBS) student, I went to HBS parties. There, I met and talked with many of the students, both male and female. The women were overwhelmingly competent, aggressive, unemotional, confident, levelheaded, and objective. HBS, after all, virtually requires these characteristics for admission.

Scholastically, the women did very well. However, socially, they had a harder time. Over and over I heard the men complaining that the HBS women were "more masculine than men," "ball breakers," and "dogs" (totally untrue, assuming they meant unattractive). One man told me, point-blank, that one couldn't possibly go out with women at the school because they weren't "really women."

They certainly looked like women to me. In fact, every one I met conformed to feminine prescriptions of appearance much more closely than I. They wore distinctly "women's" clothing to classes and sexy ball gowns to the big parties. They wore makeup. They shaved their legs. In short, they followed all the rules but one—and were rejected for being "too masculine" or, perhaps, too much like "businessmen."

In *The Cinderella Complex*, Colette Dowling describes a similar source of conflict for women. Beginning with fairy tales, we've been taught to see women as helpless, troubled creatures who are "saved" or "swept off their feet" by gallant and capable young men. We're taught that men are motivated to save women because of their beauty and helplessness. Consequently, we may imagine ourselves as helpless and needy, waiting for a man to save us from loneliness and unhappiness.

The basic Cinderella theme is still captivating the hearts of millions of people, many of them adults. The film *An Officer and a Gentleman*, for instance, is a popular 1980s version of the same tale. In this film, the hero is a young naval cadet who has decided to escape from poverty by becoming a navy pilot. He falls in love with one of the many local factory workers who would like to marry a successful cadet. At one point in the movie, our hero asks his girlfriend why, if she wants to leave her home so much, she doesn't become a cadet herself. She doesn't answer. Her apparent assumption is that she couldn't or shouldn't have to do it. The film ends with our hero walking into the factory and literally carrying our modern Cinderella away. The audience responds to his white uniform, his (traditional) attractiveness, the background music, and all the factory workers' applause and cheers.

Do we really believe this myth and apply it to our lives? Dowling presents evidence that many women do just that. She argues that we want and expect men to take care of us and instill our lives with meaning and purpose.[4] And regardless of whether or not we get our wish, we often feel helpless and dependent.

How do we feel about ourselves if we feel unable to deal with the world on our own? How do we feel if we believe that only a man can validate our existence? We feel a painful lack of self-efficacy, and our self-esteem is unstable and low—underlying characteristics of people who develop diet/weight preoccupation and eating disorders. From this basis of helplessness and low self-esteem, we are drawn to the images of thin, "beautiful" women who seem to have their pick of interested men and, thus, are supposedly happy, safe, and respected.

And what happens when we "fall in love"? If you can believe the fairy tale, we "live happily ever after." As simple as that. Unfortunately, a great many of us are disappointed. We are waiting for myths to come true. We are waiting to fall in love. We hope love will arrive and stay, instead of seeking and developing it actively. We make ourselves as "beautiful" as we can and then wait for our "other half" instead of working to feel whole and developing a variety of supportive relationships. And once married, many couples fail to put the essential work into creating a lasting relationship, partly because they didn't know that any work was needed.

The modern value that divorce is a reasonable and respectable way to solve marital problems has also added to the lack of control we so often feel. Not long ago, women could feel confident that, once married, they would stay married, because divorce was relatively unusual. Today, we are very much aware that nothing is certain.

If a married woman does not have the training or experience to support herself, then she is, in fact, justified in feeling very much at risk and out of control. As women get older, they see many of their friends getting divorced, becoming instantly impoverished, and very often *not* receiving the child support granted by the court. A great many middle-aged men choose to date and later remarry younger women. Hence, the older a woman is, the smaller her chances of marrying should she want to do so. This relatively modern source of insecurity can add to feelings of inadequacy and of being out of control of one's future.

Last, but not least, there has been a lot of talk about sexual "equality" and the new opportunity for women to succeed in traditionally male spheres. Significant progress *has* been made. But the reality is that sexism is still flourishing in the U.S. of A. Our society still grants economic, political, and interpersonal power to men. Our society still refuses to grant women equal rights in its Constitu-

tion. Our society still expects women to do most of the unpaid and low-paid labor. And our society still considers women "less competent" than men.[5]

As if this weren't bad enough, we have all heard denials that sexism is a major stumbling block. Women who have succeeded against the odds are held up as "proof" that discrimination is no longer a problem. Thus we are left experiencing sexism but being told that it's insignificant. It seems that only our own shortcomings and our own lack of control are left to blame.

In short, the modern world is a very confusing, internally inconsistent, and scary place to live. We have all been taught values and expectations that conflict with each other and with our basic human needs. Since we internalize these values, we feel pressured to meet conflicting demands from within and without. Consequently, there is often no way to "win," and we feel out of control and inadequate.

What is the solution? Certainly not weight loss! Our bodies are acting as scapegoats. We have implicitly agreed to focus on them instead of looking at more profound areas of our lives, but we can change this unwritten and unspoken "agreement." No *simple* solution exists; however, we can strive to reject destructive values and embrace a supportive set of values. For instance, we can reject the idea that women should be "feminine" and men should be "masculine." Instead, we can accept that all people need the freedom to express all aspects of themselves (the so-called feminine *and* masculine aspects).

We have evidence that this is both possible and helpful. Femininity and masculinity are not two poles, but the two ends of a continuum. Few people are completely masculine or feminine; however, women are trained to tend toward the feminine end of the continuum and men to tend toward the masculine end. Those who lie toward the center of this continuum are androgynous—both masculine and feminine. Studies indicate that femininity correlates with the lowest levels of self-esteem, masculinity correlates with higher levels of self-esteem, and *androgyny correlates with the highest levels of self-esteem.*[6]

Why? At least in part because androgynous people have rejected destructive societal norms and taken more control over their personal development. They have freed themselves from sex-role prescriptions. They can be whoever they want to be. From that position of personal freedom and strength, people naturally feel better about themselves.

Both men and women can reject traditional roles and thus overcome the no-win nature of old prescriptions. If we reject damaging sex-role stereotypes, both consciously and unconsciously, we will no longer try to conform to them. This process is difficult to carry out because we habitually refer to destructive values as though they were "true." Even after making a decision to reject these values, they may continue to influence our behavior and feelings. However, efforts to "work through" problematic assumptions and expectations are well spent. In order to understand ourselves and progress, we need to know what's driving us.

Even after we manage to let go of harmful prescriptions, our work will not be finished. Many people (and the media) will continue to pressure us to conform to social norms rather than allow us to choose freely. *Everyone is comfortable if we try to improve our lives through a weight-loss program; but as soon as*

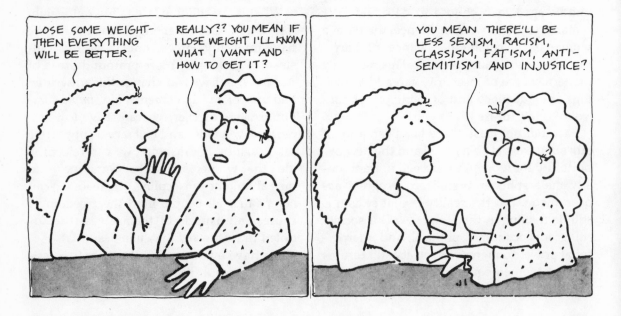

we try to improve our lives by choosing atypical values and goals, people start becoming uncomfortable. The seemingly "personal" goals of self-development and improvement become *political* in nature.

How so? If people stop making choices based on traditional sex roles, the consequences will be extensive. Women will become more powerful, and will insist upon an egalitarian society. That spells CHANGE. It is not surprising that there is so much resistance to egalitarian values, for people are terrified by change. In a society where it seems that there is not enough love or material goods to go around, people cling to traditional values whether those values are inequitable and irrational or not.

This process of personal and social change is essential to our struggle for freedom from diet/weight conflict. As long as we suffer from feelings of helplessness, inadequacy, and low self-esteem, we will feel *compelled* to increase our self-worth. If we see diet and weight control as the best way to increase our value and personal power, and hence boost our self-esteem, we will struggle for that. If we believe that only passive, weak women get "Prince Charming," then we'll wait around, hoping, and feeling out of control. If we expect men to instill our lives with meaning and purpose, then we will fail to take the necessary steps to find meaning and purpose on our own.

We have better options. For instance, if you are passively waiting for "Mr. or Ms. Right" to come along and save you—stop waiting! You require loving relationships *right now*, not when some person magically appears. You also need to take an active, assertive role in your own life. You cannot fulfill your needs *and* conform to a passive social image.

If you are struggling to be underweight (according to your own body's standards),

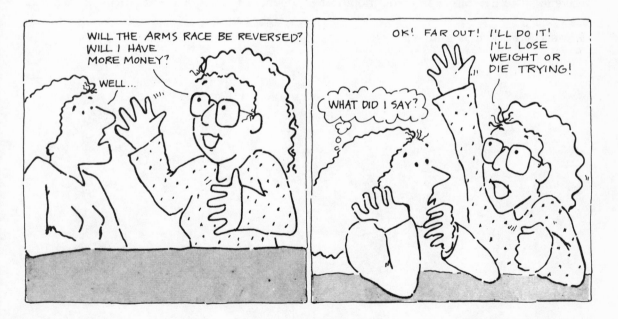

Sorting Out Our Values

then you are trying to conform to an aesthetic value that conflicts with your physical well-being. Of course you feel inadequate and helpless! You have accepted an impossible position. You cannot fulfill your body's demands *and* conform to that destructive aesthetic value. No matter what you do, you will feel dissatisfied, and you will blame yourself for it. Choose to stop! Instead, accept, love, and enjoy your body as it was meant to be. *Then* you can redirect that formerly wasted energy to work on things that really matter.

Most of us have not been taught to question, select, and create our own values and life-styles. Instead, we have been taught to absorb, mimic, and accept. We need to carve out consistent values and goals that support, rather than thwart, our quest for personal fulfillment. And, of course, this cannot be accomplished in a day, or a week, or a year. It has to be an ongoing process that helps us move in a positive direction throughout our lives.

Those who sell weight-reduction programs claim that weight loss will improve just about every aspect of our lives: our health, our relationships, our work. . . . Some people do feel better about themselves after losing weight. However, many people lose weight only to wake up to "the bare bones of their own [feelings of] inadequacy."[7] In other words, they realize that despite their thinner bodies they are still the same people, suffering from nearly all of the same problems. Weight loss has *not* transformed them into better or happier people; it has not made them more capable or successful; and it has not magically created better relationships. In fact, weight loss may have transformed them into hungry, tense, and irritable people who see the world as a colorless and unfriendly place.

It is far more likely that the kind of personal work suggested in this chapter will improve the quality of your life. Give it at least as much time and energy as you have devoted to programs that focus on diet and weight control.

PERSONAL QUESTIONS:
FIGURING OUT WHAT REALLY MATTERS

We are faced with a difficult task: to reject destructive values, embrace constructive values, and think up new values that are missing. In order to do these things, we have to sort through the values that pressure us from without, sort through the values we have already absorbed (that pressure us from within), and select the best possible group. We must develop a personal philosophy of life.

By personal philosophy, I mean a group of ideas that guide your behavior. It is not an abstract set of ideas that have little bearing on your life. You already have a philosophy of life (which you continually apply) even if you've never thought about its content. As you begin to explore your values—what really matters to you, what you really want, and why—you will be in the process of discovering your existing philosophy. Perhaps you will discover that parts of it are harmful and will want to make changes. In any case, it is completely *yours*, to create, change, and use as you like.

As you work through the following questions and exercises, remind yourself: you deserve unconditional self-acceptance and respect. Furthermore, you can explore and grow more readily if you accept yourself on an unconditional basis. You want to change something about yourself? Good! That shows you are looking for (and finding) ways to progress. It does not change the fact that you are perfectly fine as you are.

If you are forever feeling disorganized or suffer from chronic procrastination, make a daily plan of what you would like to accomplish, prioritize that list, and then make a constant effort to *do the most important first* throughout each day. This thought is the key to using your time well: "I will do the most important thing now."[8] If you would like to use your time more efficiently and/or keep sight of your goals more consistently, try using a time-management program (see Resources, p. 242).

Many of the people in my workshops are *overplanners* rather than underplanners—not in terms of their long-range plans and goals, but in terms of their daily activities. They are forever making lists of what they need to do and organizing their belongings and schedules. Consequently, they lose spontaneity and tend to focus on everything *except* the present (moment and activity). Dissatisfaction is then inevitable.

Do you draw up schedules that include daily routines *you would do automatically anyway?* Do you draw up lists or plans that you never use or that never had a purpose you can identify? If so, you need to figure out what you are really looking to control and direct. Is it your daily activities or is it something else? Compulsive planning, like compulsive dieting, can be a way of grasping for direction and control—a kind of direction and control that cannot be attained through organizing, planning, or dieting.

Sorting Out Our Values

RELATIONSHIPS

We all want and need loving relationships with other people. We each have our own feelings and ideas about the importance and purpose of various relationships, as well as different expectations of ourselves and other people. These are extremely important issues to explore because satisfactory relationships with other people are essential to a satisfying life.

1.   To what extent do you view a relationship as a "given"—the nature and destiny of which is outside your control—and to what extent do you view a relationship as a product of your own making? Why?

2.   Describe a network of family and friends that you would like to have now, and one you would like to have in ten years. How important are these networks and why?

3.   How often do you find yourself alone when you would rather not be alone? If this is a problem, what can you do about it?

4. How often do you find yourself with people when you would rather be alone? If this is a problem, what can you do about it?

5. What would you like to gain from friendships? Do you tend to confide in your friends and provide emotional support for one another, or do you tend to share activities and leave it at that?

6. In general, are you happy with the nature of your friendships? What would you like to change, and what would you like to keep the same?

7. Do you feel comfortable in social gatherings? Do you usually enjoy yourself? If not, why? How might you be able to enjoy yourself more?

8.   Would you like to improve your interpersonal skills? Why or why not? If you answered "yes," how important are these skills? How can you begin to improve them?

9.   What percent of your time and energy do you feel you should devote to relationships? Are you presently devoting more, less, or an optimal amount of time and energy?

10.   Do you want to have a central love relationship? If so, consider the following:

- What do you expect and want to gain from that relationship?

- Are your expectations realistic?

- Do you want your central relationship to affect your other relationships, and if so, how and why?

- What mutual goals or interests, if any, do you want to share with this person? Why?

- To what extent and in what ways do you want to be independent versus interdependent? Why?

- Are you presently seeking this person? If so, how?

11.   Use the following spaces to describe your relationship with a "significant other" (relative, friend, or co-worker). Under his/her name, describe: (a) the current nature of your relationship with that person, including problems; (b) how much time you usually spend with that person; (c) how you would like your relationship to be; and (d) steps you can take toward developing (or maintaining) your relationship as desired. Repeat this exercise on paper for other relationships that warrant thought and energy.

Name:
Current Relationship:

Time spent together per _____ = _____
Potential relationship—desired change:

Steps toward desired relationship:

PAST LESSONS—PRESENT BELIEFS

1. What personal limitations were you taught? (In other words, what were you taught you could do, and what were you taught you could not do?) How do those lessons affect you now?

2. Do you feel that you are responsible for developing a satisfying life, or do you feel as though someone or something else is supposed to provide it?

3. With whom have you experienced the most conflict?

4.   Pretend that you are the person you named in question 3. Imagine that you grew up in the same circumstances as that person, and you now think like him/her and feel what she/he feels. Complete the following sentence as if you were that person writing about yourself.

Of all the things I would like to see _____ (your own name)
do, I would *most* like her to _____ .
I'm really glad that she _____ ,
but I *really* wish that she would stop _____ .
All I really want is for her to be _____ , but sometimes I
wonder if _____ .
I think that _____
_____ .

5.   Now go back to being *yourself* and complete the following sentences.

Of all the things I want to do, I *most* want to _____ .
I'm really glad that I _____ ,
but I *really* wish I would stop _____ .
All I really want is _____ , but sometimes I wonder if
_____ .
I think that _____
_____ .

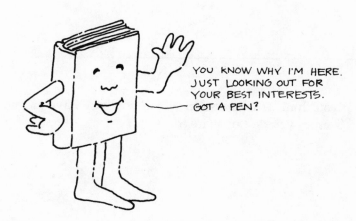

YOU KNOW WHY I'M HERE.
JUST LOOKING OUT FOR
YOUR BEST INTERESTS.
GOT A PEN?

Sorting Out Our Values

6. Make a list of all the differences and similarities between your values and the values of the person you named in question 3.

VALUES YOU SHARE	VALUES YOU DO NOT SHARE

7. Can you think of instances in which you may have judged yourself according to some of these "values you do not share"?

USING TIME: MAKING CHOICES, SETTING GOALS

How you spend your time is vital to who you are. Your life is your time: it is all the minutes, hours, and days, strung out in a continuous line, that go by no matter what else happens. If you do not value your time, then you do not value your life. Do you respect your time? If you spend your time in ways you do not enjoy, then you will want time to pass quickly. If you set limits on what you can do or how you can act (until you lose weight, for instance), then you will focus on the future instead of living fully in the present.

Do you enjoy the way you spend most of your time? Do you know why you spend it the way you do? I occasionally ask myself what I would be doing "right now" if I had only one or two years to live. If my answer is significantly different from what I am actually doing, then I see whether or not I can justify it. Do I have a good reason for postponing gratification? Am I pursuing a worthwhile goal? If not, I know that it is time to switch gears and redirect my energy.

We are all fragile. We are all going to die someday—and maybe much sooner than we expect. Even if we live to be 120, we will want to feel that we used our time well. Take a close look at the way you are spending your time. If you aren't thrilled with what you see and you do not have very good reasons for suffering with it, then you are wasting your time and thereby wasting a precious piece of your life.

1. Suppose that you had only two years to live, starting today. What would you do for the next two years?

2. Given that you (presumably) have more than two years to live, what do you plan to do for the next two years and why? How do you feel about these choices?

Sorting Out Our Values

3.   Do you tend to be too busy or not busy enough? If so, how can you achieve a better balance?

4.   Make a list of things you enjoy. This list can include recreational activities, types of achievement, foods, types of interactions, ways of helping others, etc.

ACTIVITIES AND OTHER THINGS I ENJOY

5.   Look over your list. Can you take better advantage of these sources of satisfaction? If so, how?

6. Make a list of things that *might* make you feel good if you tried them.

ACTIVITIES AND OTHER THINGS I MIGHT ENJOY

7. Look over your list. What would you like to try first? When can you begin?

8. Make a list of your personal goals. These should include goals regarding family, friends, health, mental development, travel, material desires, personal contributions to humanity, etc., that you would like to pursue in your lifetime.

Sorting Out Our Values

```
┌─────────────────────────────────────────────────────┐
│                  MY PERSONAL GOALS                  │
├─────────────────────────────────────────────────────┤
│                                                     │
│                                                     │
│                                                     │
│                                                     │
│                                                     │
│                                                     │
│                                                     │
│                                                     │
│                                                     │
└─────────────────────────────────────────────────────┘
```

9. Make a list of your professional goals. These should include desired position(s), income, impact on people and organizations, work schedules, etc., that you would like to pursue in your lifetime.

```
┌─────────────────────────────────────────────────────┐
│                MY PROFESSIONAL GOALS                │
├─────────────────────────────────────────────────────┤
│                                                     │
│                                                     │
│                                                     │
│                                                     │
│                                                     │
│                                                     │
│                                                     │
│                                                     │
│                                                     │
└─────────────────────────────────────────────────────┘
```

10. Make a list of your personal goals for this year.

MY PERSONAL GOALS FOR THIS YEAR

11. Make a list of your professional (or academic) goals for this year.

MY PROFESSIONAL GOALS FOR THIS YEAR

Sorting Out Our Values

CONCLUSION

This chapter brings up many complex issues. It outlines a lot of exercises, and it suggests lifelong examination of values and goals. These may not *seem* to bear on your diet/ weight obsession, but they do nonetheless. Once you concentrate your energy on goals of your own choosing—goals unrelated to diet and weight—you will attain some of that elusive "control" you crave. You will also be able to put diet/weight control into perspective. You will see that it truly is a small part of your life—something that affects the way you feel but *doesn't* affect your value as a person and *doesn't* "make or break" your quest for happiness.

As you make changes in your life, beware of trying to change too much too fast. Lasting change takes time. If you have trouble getting started, try making a few very minor changes. Try answering the phone differently or taking a different route to work (or school). That way you can experiment with how it feels to do something differently without taking any big risks. Even very silly experiments with change can help you move on to bigger challenges.

Most important, don't forget to get support from friends, family, and/or a therapist. I cannot overemphasize this: you need not struggle alone! In fact, struggling with serious problems in isolation often hurts instead of helps. Treat yourself with the loving concern you would afford your best friend. You wouldn't ask that she struggle all alone. Tell someone about your new expectations and hopes for yourself. Ask her to check in with you occasionally to find out about your progress and to offer support.

You are a very valuable person exactly as you are. You deserve to feel good about yourself and your life. At times, we all find it difficult to be who we want to be. But luckily, we are incredibly powerful. We can let go of the damaging lessons we have learned. We can reach beyond the fears and walls that past "hurts" have created. *We can figure out what really matters to us, and then work toward whatever we value and desire.*

> You can be anybody you want to be
> You can love whomever you will
> You can travel any country where
>   your heart leads
> And know I will love you still
> You can live by yourself
> You can gather friends around
> You can choose one special one
> And the only measure of your words
>   and your deeds
> Will be the love you leave behind
>   when you're done.
>
> Fred Small, "Everything Possible"[9]

7

EXPRESSING OUR RIGHTS AND NEEDS

We are surrounded by people who habitually say and do things that encourage diet/weight obsession and eating disorders. When people talk about their weight-loss programs, it encourages us to be obsessed about our own bodies. ("*They* think they need to lose weight. They must think I need to lose weight.") When people admiringly tell us that we've lost weight or disapprovingly announce that we've gained weight, we feel pressured to be thin. ("They obviously like me more when I'm thin. I should be thin.") When people objectify others, particularly in a fattist way, we are reminded that people are forever being judged on their appearance. Therefore, we feel pressured to look as "beautiful" as possible. ("They are judging that person on the basis of her appearance. I wonder how I measure up?")

How are we supposed to free ourselves from preoccupation when we are constantly being encouraged to be obsessed about diet

and weight? First, we can make a personal decision to choose well-being over diet/weight conflict in spite of the pressure to do the reverse. We learn to live with destructive influences by identifying what is harmful and reminding ourselves of our goals and beliefs. Second, we can encourage people around us to be actively supportive. Because they have been subjected to the same destructive messages, however, we will have to teach them how to support *us* instead of our diet/weight obsession.

How can we teach them? By example and through discussion. Behaving as you would like others to behave is helpful, but it will not be sufficient because almost everyone else and the media provide a constant stream of poor examples. You will need to educate the people around you. This does not mean aggressively attacking their behavior. It means explaining why a particular behavior is harmful and suggesting specific alternatives. Deep inside, no one wants to hurt others. If people become aware of the destructiveness of certain comments or actions, they are usually willing to act differently.

COMMON INFLUENCES WE NEED TO DISCOURAGE

Fattism

Fattism is one of the most widely accepted forms of prejudice and discrimination in our culture. Like racism and sexism, it is a prejudice based on physical characteristics. Some fattism is obvious. Direct criticism of someone's weight, for instance, is blatantly fattist. Many fattist comments, however, are not so obvious.

Suppose someone says, "My Aunt Gertrude lost forty pounds. She's at a much more reasonable weight now." The underlying (fattist) assumption is that before she lost forty pounds, her weight was "unreasonable." In reality, Aunt Gertrude may have been healthier and happier at the higher weight. Her body may have found the *loss* of those forty pounds "unreasonable."

Most people are fattist and will *defend* their fattism even if they understand that human beings naturally come in all shapes and sizes. It is very difficult to get people to stop saying and doing fattist things. They've been taught this prejudice since birth, and it is reinforced daily. Be prepared to hear certain arguments over and over.

Many people will claim that they are not fattist (and will truly believe this to be the case) but will make fattist comments under the guise of "health" and "fitness." When you point out that some people are genetically destined to be fat and hurt themselves by trying to change their natural size, they are likely to respond, "Yes, but most fat people are completely out of shape—it's unhealthy. Don't you think they should get some exercise?"

As you try to identify fattism, keep the following questions in mind. (a) Would this person criticize a stranger on the street (with disgust in her voice) because that person was smoking and thereby damaging her health? (b) Is this person disgusted by every person who has a sedentary life-style, or just by fat people who have sedentary life-styles? (c) Why is fatness so disturbing to this person —why is it worthy of comment?

Fattism can go hand in hand with a preoccupation with fitness. As people who suffer from diet/weight obsession, we usually share that preoccupation as well. Being physically active and fit can help us let go of the diet/weight obsession; therefore, I have encouraged it. But beware: as soon as fitness becomes a weight-loss technique, or a moral issue, or a way of creating and measuring personal worth, we are in trouble. If we feel that we are "bad" if we do not exercise, that is almost as harmful as feeling that we are "bad" if we are fat. Most people in our society have sedentary life-styles, but that doesn't make them bad people. It just makes them out of shape. We are all entitled to choose our own activity level, and we are worthy of respect and love regardless of how active or inactive we choose to be.

In short, overcoming fattism is a tough challenge. Even after someone seems convinced that it is unethical to be prejudiced against fat people, she is likely to return to fattist comments and arguments later. We can even find *ourselves* having fattist thoughts and feelings, despite our best efforts to reject that prejudice. We have internalized the fattism we have been taught, and society continues to brainwash us from the outside. However, we can contradict those thoughts by saying to ourselves, "There's that fattism again! I don't believe it anymore, and I won't listen to it." Those who still hold on to their fattism, on the other hand, will try to justify and disguise it. We can help them reject fattism, too.

Objectification

Our society values appearance, especially women's appearance, far too much. We are often judged, and we often judge others, solely or primarily on the basis of appearance. We often see ourselves and others treated as aesthetic objects instead of human beings. The combination of objectification and the exclusive idealization of slenderness creates tremendous pressure to be as "thin and beautiful" as possible, which in turn encourages our preoccupation.

All of us participate in this appearance mania. We are always saying that such-and-such a person "looked really great," as if appearance were a tremendously significant index to her value. Noticing and talking about appearance is not inherently harmful; however, *very frequent* comments about anything imply that it is very important. We are part of a vicious cycle: we comment on appearance frequently because we live in an appearance-conscious society; our frequent comments then encourage this appearance consciousness. Perhaps if we talk about appearance less frequently, we will stop inflating its importance.

At the very least it would be helpful if people would talk about appearance less than they talk about other characteristics such as personality and well-being. When someone mentions that they saw a mutual acquaintance and tells you little or nothing about that person except how she looked, ask for more significant news about her. Don't perpetuate the implied judgment that appearance is the most significant aspect of a human being.

Other "do nots" include spending large amounts of time looking in the mirror, criticizing your appearance, allowing yourself to be objectified or objectifying others by whistling or leering, and rating people's appearance on a scale of one to ten. Explain to other people why such behavior is harmful, and interrupt yourself when you fall into those patterns. Remember that when people are treated as aesthetic objects instead of as human beings, they are encouraged to treat themselves as objects and to feel like objects. Aesthetic objects such as paintings and sculpture have little to offer beyond their appearance—not so with human beings. We need to act, and to encourage others to act, as though we all believe it.

Weight-Reduction Propaganda

We all hear a constant drone of commercials that tell us to improve ourselves and our lives by losing weight. The underlying assumptions of these commercials are that weight loss is "good" and improves the quality of life, that weight-loss dieting is "good," that those who lose weight are "good," and that thin people are happier and better adjusted than fat people. Thus, we are encouraged to feel that we should be thin, more or less regardless of cost.

It is virtually impossible to avoid hearing and seeing these commercials; however, we can either ignore them or criticize them. We must learn to ignore them in order to protect our new outlook. We need to criticize them in order to remind ourselves and others of their destructive influence and thus ensure that we do not passively (and unconsciously) accept their messages.

Unfortunately, the people around us accept these messages. We are faced with a stream of conversations about weight, food, and weight-loss programs. In order to attain freedom from our preoccupation, we need to redirect or walk away from these destructive conversations.

BUILDING ALLIES
FOR FREEDOM

If we initiate a serious discussion every time someone says or does something that supports diet/weight conflict, we will drive everyone, including ourselves, crazy. There are an infinite variety of ways to contradict harmful messages, ranging from serious discussion to lighthearted disagreement, to avoiding the subject completely. Try out all different ways of making your point. Try a serious discussion of the facts about diet and weight. Try jokingly telling your fattist friend that, yes, if she gains even one pound you will hate her forever and her life will be over. And try simply changing the subject.

We cannot teach every person we meet to stop supporting diet/weight conflict; however, if we teach our closest friends and relatives, we will have done ourselves and others a great service.

I cannot overemphasize the effect of loved ones' attitudes and behavior. If loved ones encourage your preoccupation (whether they mean to or not), you will find it much more difficult to free yourself. Luckily, those who love you should be most willing to be supportive rather than destructive. Through honest discussion, and by sharing this book, you can encourage the people around you to be your best allies. But be diplomatic. Remember that they were (and are still) subjected to the same insidious lessons that have led you to be preoccupied with diet and weight. Explosions of anger and frustration are counterproductive. You need to see friends and relatives understanding and supporting you, not defending themselves against critical attacks.

Most important, be patient. Almost everyone supports the development and maintenance of diet/weight conflict and eating disorders without knowing it. We have been trained to do so. Even after we understand many aspects of the problem and begin to try to undermine diet/weight conflict, we can slip into destructive behavior. After all, objectifying others, making fattist comments, and talking about diet and weight control are considered normal. Everyone (including you and me) needs understanding, time, and practice in order to stop encouraging this preoccupation.

Example 1

Suppose that a friend of yours has just begun to talk about her latest weight-loss diet. She seems to want to swap frustrations, stories, and advice, and she assumes that you are the perfect friend for this purpose. What could you do?

You could treat this as a good opportunity to discuss your new thoughts and feelings about diet and weight. This friend will probably be interested in the physiological mechanisms with which she has been fighting. First, you could discuss the effects of dieting and setpoint theory with her. Next, you might want to discuss your preoccupation and find out whether or not your friend has a similar problem. You can explain to her that weight-loss programs (and the assumption that weight loss is a positive goal) support the preoccupation you are trying to overcome. Ideally, this friend could become a valuable ally who, like you, will work toward freedom from diet/weight preoccupation. At the very least, she could agree to stop undermining your efforts.

Example 2

Suppose a friend of yours notices an obese man on the street and says, "Look at that, isn't it disgusting?" What could you say?

My instinctive reply is, "No 'it' isn't, and the person you just insulted isn't an it—he's a human being!" Unfortunately, this type of reply tends to initiate an angry confrontation rather than a helpful discussion. As soon as we attack someone, all her defenses go up and little is likely to be accomplished. Many

alternatives are possible depending on the circumstances. For instance: "I know you didn't *mean* any harm, but I find that comment very hurtful." (Then you can talk about fattism, its prevalence, and your feelings about it.) Or try one of my workshop participant's suggestions: "I wonder who's inside? Don't you?"

Example 3

Suppose your mother is a chronic dieter with whom you have shared many weight-loss regimens. She pressures you to be thin just as she pressures herself to be thin, and the shared frustrations of chronic dieting have become a big part of your relationship. How can you break out of this destructive pattern without losing closeness and intimacy?

In many cases, a private discussion can help. Whether you live with your mother or see her twice a year, you can probably improve your relationship through honest and loving discussions. Try starting with the love. When was the last time you told your mother how much you love and respect her? (Not only does she need to know it, she needs to hear it now and then.) Have you ever told her what you particularly appreciate about her or acknowledged how hard she has tried? Start by appreciating your mother, then discuss how you are hurting each other (without meaning to).

Share some of the changes you're going through. Explain your current struggle toward freedom from the diet/weight obsession and explain your greatest fears. Are you afraid of losing your closeness? Are you afraid of losing her respect and love? Are you afraid of hurting her? After expressing your love, respect, and fear, you will have paved the way to ask for her help. For instance, you could ask her to stop commenting on your weight and diet. You could ask to share conversations and activities other than (and instead of) diet and weight concerns. Make it clear that you are not rejecting her. If you can express your love, respect, and desire for closeness, she'll be more likely to understand and accept why you are no longer willing to discuss or worry about calories, weight, etc.

I've made this sound easy when it is, in fact, difficult. Immediate family members are almost always involved in the development and maintenance of the diet/weight obsession, and they are almost always the hardest to influence. The extent to which you will need to deal with them directly depends on your situation. The extent to which you will be able to improve those relationships depends, in part, on your personal strength and flexibility (and theirs). Try to set realistic goals.

Most important, always remember that *you don't have to change anyone else's behavior in order to benefit:* just explaining your position and needs can help you regardless of how they react. At the very least, you can feel good about asserting yourself. You may even discover something about yourself. The influence of those who are close to you is probably the strongest *inside your own head.* As you confront their destructive behavior, you may free yourself of some destructive thoughts and feelings.

Assertiveness

If you feel that you cannot stand up for your rights and needs, ask yourself why you feel that way. Do you often swallow your opinions and feelings because you don't think you deserve attention, or because you don't want to "rock the boat," or because you are afraid that someone will disapprove? Many people—especially women—are not assertive, and frequently the problem goes hand in hand with low self-esteem. Becoming more assertive is very important as you work toward freedom from your diet/weight obsession.

Why is it difficult for many of us to stand up for what we need and believe? One reason is that we don't think we deserve to have our needs met. Which of your parents seemed to be valued most in your household? Whose needs were met (or thoughts heard) most often? If we have learned that we are not worthy of standing up for ourselves, we must unlearn it. We all deserve to be heard. We all have something worthwhile to say. And we all deserve to have our needs met.

Another reason why we do not stand up for ourselves is that we don't think we can do so successfully. We fear that if we make a demand or point out the harmfulness of others' behavior, they will become offended or angry and refuse to respond in a helpful way.

In order to speak out, we need to know that if people respond with anger or disapproval, we won't crumple up and die, nor feel that we did something wrong. We also need to know *how* to assert ourselves—how to be *as-*

sertive instead of aggressive or passive. Most of us can benefit from books on assertiveness (see Resources, pp. 240-242) or an assertiveness training course. In addition, we can improve our skills for dealing with conflict.

INGREDIENTS OF A DISARMING AND EFFECTIVE RESPONSE

We need skills in order to respond when someone mistreats us; when we see someone behaving destructively and we want to make her aware of the harm done; and when we want someone to do something (e.g., go somewhere or agree with us) and she is resisting.

When we are in need of a disarming and effective reply, we are often in a situation where someone has hurt or offended us. If this is the case, we have a decision to make. Do we want to strike back and hurt this person—vent our frustration and pain on a seemingly deserving target? Or would we rather let go of our desire for revenge and encourage this person to change her objectionable behavior? The first option is quite easy to carry out but gets us nowhere.

The most important thing to remember in the face of conflict is that people need to know you're on their side. They need to know that you respect their opinions and feelings. Once you allow them a little time and emotional separation from their behavior and show them respect, you can say much more without triggering their defenses.

The steps described below may seem drawn out and cumbersome. "It would take forever!" you might complain. This method *is* more time-consuming than most people's instinctive method of handling conflict, but that is what it takes to get good results. People are fragile. It's easy to threaten and hurt one another. Consequently, it takes time and patience to deal with conflict in a nonthreatening, disarming, and effective way.

Here is an overview of the steps:

1. Identify (clarify and restate) her viewpoint.
2. Get your interpretation confirmed.
3. Isolate each point of disagreement.
4. Point out how you agree.
5. State your point of view.
6. Get your viewpoint confirmed.

Some of the steps can be compressed or skipped, depending on the situation, how well you know the person involved, how much she trusts and respects you, and whether or not she feels that you trust and respect her. But beware of too many shortcuts. If you find yourself replacing steps 1–4 with "Yes, but . . ." you've gone too far. In the face of a disagreement, even people you know well need to be reassured that you are listening, and that you respect their opinion.

Step 1: Identify (Clarify and Restate) Her Viewpoint

Restate the other person's view in order to (a) make sure that you understand the conflict, (b) show that you listened to and understood her, and (c) show that you care about and respect her opinion.

EXAMPLES:

> "Hmmm . . . I think I understand what you're saying. You think that . . ."

> "I'm not sure if I understand what you're trying to say; do you mean . . . ?"

> "Are you saying that . . . ?"

Step 2: Get Your Interpretation Confirmed

Unless the person confirms your understanding of her opinion, you leave yourself open to a frustrating experience: you provide a brilliant response, she then agrees with your viewpoint, but instead of changing her point of view or behavior, she presents you with a new objection. "Oh, I didn't say that! I meant . . ." Sound familiar?

It is easy to ask for confirmation. Just end your statements with a question such as "Is that what you meant?" or "Did I get that right?" If she rejects your interpretation, fine. You know that you needed to probe in order to fully understand the problem, and the other person will appreciate your attempts to understand. Ask for *and listen to* the new explanation and then try again: restate her viewpoint and ask for confirmation.

In the process of making sure that you understand the other person's viewpoint, you may discover that you do not stand in conflict after all. (You may even change your point of view!) Some people automatically assume their opinion is right and just go through the *motions* of identifying the other person's point of view. That may be an inappropriate concern at this point, but skilled debaters are famous for being able to "win" arguments regardless of whether they're right or wrong. Once *you* become a skilled debater, be sure to avoid this unkind and irresponsible behavior.

Step 3: Isolate Each Point of Disagreement

In the face of conflict, you need to know exactly what you're up against. Ideally, you would like the person to say that she has only one point of disagreement. Then you know that if you overcome that objection, you'll be home free. Unless you isolate the disagreement, you invite a common and frustrating experience: you answer the original objection only to be presented with another objection. (For example, "You know, I think you're right about that, but I *also* think that . . .") Of course, people can respond that way even if you have isolated the objection, but they will do so less frequently.

EXAMPLES

> "Do you think that if it weren't for . . . (the objection), you would feel (or act) differently?"

> "Is the only reason why you . . . (the opposing view or behavior), because . . . (the objection)?"

> "It looks like we would be in complete agreement if it weren't for . . . (the objection) and . . . (a second objection). Is that right?"

Step 4: Point Out How You Agree

This can be a difficult step because you strongly disagree with the person in at least one area; however, you can usually find some common ground. For instance, you may not agree with someone's actions or statements, yet appreciate her *intentions*. Or you may agree about the importance of the subject. In any case, it is crucial that you *agree with the person in some way before you go on to express your point of view*. Why? Because in order to do so effectively, you need to be on the same side of the fence. You need to show that you are not against her.

EXAMPLES

"I can see why you feel that way. You . . . (explain why she feels as she does). Is that right?"

"You know, I think you're right. If I were you, I might say the same thing because . . ."

"I think I understand what you mean. I once . . . (tell an anecdote that illustrates her viewpoint in a favorable way)."

"You know, I really appreciate your intentions. It appears that you . . . (objectionable belief or action) because you really care about . . . (person or concept involved)."

Step 5: State Your Point of View

Now you have paved the way to express your thoughts and feelings. Try to express yourself clearly and firmly, but not aggressively. Say whatever you have to say as though you are sure that the other person is going to understand and agree with you— almost as though no disagreement exists. Do not attack the person to whom you are speaking. Wherever possible, criticize behavior or statements rather than the person; and, wherever possible, allow that person to gain distance from her behavior before using negative words such as "unjust," "fattist," "cruel," or "sexist" (or avoid such words altogether).

If your viewpoint is somewhat long and involved, try asking if she understands what you're saying along the way. Even if she doesn't agree, at least you'll know she is understanding your point.

Step 6: Get Your Viewpoint Confirmed

Ideally, you would like the other person to be able to summarize what you've said in her own words and agree. This may be a lot to strive for, but try to assume that it will happen as you speak. (If you can convince yourself that it's bound to happen, you will be more relaxed and effective.) When a person seems unconvinced, try to get her to explain *your* point of view to you. This will give you a chance to correct any misinterpretation and improve the other person's understanding. (Not to mention that any point of view will probably sound more reasonable to the person when explained in her own words and voice.)

"Do you understand why I feel this way?"

"Do you see what I mean?"

"Do you understand what I'm saying, or would you like me to clarify something?"

If the person says she understands but actually seems confused, try saying something

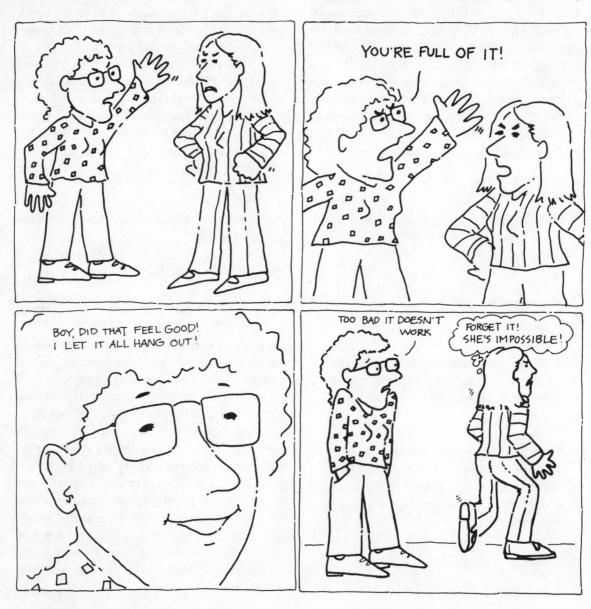

like, "You do? Great. Would you mind repeating that back to me? I'm not sure if I explained it right." If the person says she understands but then states the same objection over again (which you just answered), try something like, "Hmm . . . I think I know just what you mean, but I don't see how it differs from what you said before. Could you explain it to me?"

Ineffective Phrases to Avoid

"Yes, but . . ." Whenever you reply with "Yes, but . . ." you convey the following message (even though you may not mean to): "That last statement was so worthless that I'm going to dismiss it with a quick 'Yes, but . . .' and move right on to *my* point of view. So—listen and learn from one who knows better." People don't appreciate that message. It encourages them to react defensively, and it sets you up on opposite sides.

"You're wrong!" This statement strengthens the other person's conviction because it suggests that you are insensitive and close-minded. It also tends to elicit anger, resentment, and stubbornness.

"How can you say that?" This suggests that you don't respect the other person, so she becomes defensive. "Obviously," she thinks, "I just open my mouth and speak—who are *you* to criticize what I say?"

"You're so . . . (negative adjective)." Name-calling, of course, is the antithesis of a disarming and effective response. If you find yourself reduced to that, apologize and start over.

Very Effective Phrases to Use

"Maybe you can help me out . . ." People love to help. They love knowing that they have something to offer someone else, and that someone else would trust and respect them enough to ask. By enlisting their help, you can circumvent their defenses and "team up" with them. Teammates are much more cooperative than opponents. As soon as they agree to help you, they implicitly agree to try to understand your point of view.

"Would you mind if I told you something personal?" People hate to be *told* to listen; however, we all love to be confided in and trusted. If you seem to trust others to listen in an empathetic way, they are likely to try to live up to that expectation.

"What was that like for you?" People like (and need) to talk about how they have felt and how they feel. If you draw out their reactions and feelings, they will usually want to hear your reactions and feelings, too. As you show concern for each other, it will be much easier to understand and resolve any disagreement.

"I'm very interested in your opinion." This statement explicitly assures people that you are willing to listen and learn, even though you may disagree. It puts you and the other person on the same side.

"Tell me more." If you encourage people to talk and then listen to them, they will be more likely to trust and listen to you.

"I appreciate the way you've listened to me." It's always helpful to appreciate people's efforts, especially when they have behaved in a way you value highly. When you appreciate that someone has listened to you, she will probably appreciate that you, too, listened well. In any case, open appreciation almost always makes both people feel good.

An Example of the Method in Use

Participants in my workshops often describe how their parents or employers have pressured them to "improve" their appearance by losing weight or wearing makeup. Most of them report that they dealt with this criticism and pressure by trying to conform, or by ignoring it (and therefore hearing more about it later). Either way, they lost. They felt abused and pressured to obsess about their diet, weight, and appearance, and they saw no way to resist that pressure. Here is a woman choosing a different option.

Janet is a secretary who is being reviewed by her boss, Margaret.

Margaret: ". . . in short, Janet, your performance has been better than ever this year, and I'm very pleased.

"Now I want to touch on something I'm concerned about. I've noticed that your appearance has changed for the worse: you've gained weight, you don't wear makeup any more, and often you wear the most, well, you wear rather unattractive clothing. I get the feeling that you're depressed, that you don't like yourself, and that that's why you don't take care of yourself.

"In a way this is your own business. But you're the person people see before they get to me, and, consequently, your appearance reflects on me. Do you understand? I'm very concerned about the appearance of the office, and I'm con-

cerned about you as a person. Is something wrong?"

(The phone rings with a call for Margaret. She talks for a while and then hangs up.)

"Sorry about the interruption. I'm so pressed for time these days, it's crazy. . . . Where were we?"

Janet: "Well, you just asked me if something was wrong. . . . But you seem so busy. Do you have fifteen minutes or so to discuss this, or would you rather plan to talk another time?"

Margaret: "We can talk about it now. My meeting doesn't start for another half hour."

Janet: "Okay, good. . . . Let me make sure that I understand what you're saying. You worry that I'm feeling bad about myself, and you're feeling that I don't make myself attractive enough to fulfill my responsibility as your secretary. Is that right?"

Margaret: "Oh no! You fulfill your secretarial responsibilities very, very well. It would be virtually impossible for me to replace you. But yes, I'm concerned about you and the way you present yourself. I think it would be better for you, as well as for the image of our office, if you would take better care of yourself."

Janet: "I really appreciate your concern. You've always been very good to me. But since this is my annual review, I want to make sure I understand the problem completely. If I felt good about myself, and I took care of myself, would you be completely satisfied with my performance?"

Margaret: "Yes."

Janet: "Would you mind if I told you something personal? Since you're concerned, I really want you to understand."

Margaret: "Yes, please do, dear."

Janet: "It's true that when I started to work here I was thinner and I wore makeup and different clothes. I guess that most people saw me as you did—a very well-groomed and cheerful woman. In reality, though, I wasn't all that happy and I was insecure. I was completely obsessed with my appearance—I felt I always had to look exactly right. Looking that way cost me a lot. I was always on a semistarvation diet. I spent a lot of time making sure that every hair was in place and that my makeup was perfect. I have severe skin problems, and my dermatologist said that I shouldn't wear makeup. But I ignored him because my appearance was more important to me than my skin or my health. I really tortured myself to look good. Do you know what I mean?"

Margaret: "Yes! I know exactly what you mean, but don't you think . . ."

Janet: "Wait. I'm sorry to interrupt you, but I need to finish my train of thought. It's not easy for me to explain all this, but I'd like to finish. Okay?"

Margaret: "Sorry—go ahead."

Janet: "One of the reasons why I was so obsessed with my appearance was that I *didn't* like myself. I was always trying to make up for my inadequacies by looking as attractive as possible. I wasn't comfortable in those clothes because they were too tight and restrictive. And I wasn't comfortable—I didn't feel good—at that weight. Makeup was also a bad thing for me, not only because of my skin problem but because I was trying to make myself look like a model instead of accepting and appreciating my own face. It's only now that I feel better about myself that I've been able to treat myself *better:* by eating when I'm hungry instead of starving myself all the time, by wearing more comfortable clothing, and by taking good care of my skin.

"I know that you're trying to help me, not trying to hurt me, that's why I'm telling you all this. Since you're concerned, I want you to know that I feel better about myself now than I did before. I finally feel like I'm okay just as I am. I think that's one of the reasons why I've gotten better at my job over the last year. I'm a lot more comfortable with myself. I feel more confident. Now you're telling me that I'm *not* okay as I am: that I have to lose weight and wear makeup and uncomfortable clothing. If I have to do it for the 'office image,' that's one thing, and you're right to tell me so. But as far as my *own* good is concerned—that's something else. Do you see that what you're asking will hurt instead of help me?"

Margaret: "I think I do. But does looking unkempt help you feel better about yourself? Because I can't believe it does, and it's a problem."

Janet: "Do I really look 'unkempt'?"

Margaret: "Well, yes. I guess the main problem is that your hair tends to look uncombed and your clothes are too casual."

Janet: "I'm really sorry. I didn't mean to look messy. I guess that my hair gets windblown when I walk to work. If I wear more formal clothing and comb my hair when I get here, will you be satisfied?"

Margaret: "Yes, I'm sure that will be fine."

This example may sound unrealistic (partly because bosses are rarely that sensitive and partly because few people can explain themselves that well under pressure), but it provides the general idea. Don't feel bad if you have trouble producing disarming and effective responses—it's not easy! But be assured that practice helps. Where you once would have been speechless with anger and pain, you can learn to think of something to say. At first you won't be able to remember what to do. You may lose your train of thought or your temper; you may get confused by a good debater; and you may not say what you mean to say. But the more you practice, the better you'll be able to stand up for yourself. Your efforts will be well spent. For if you can learn to deal with conflict well, your confidence, self-esteem, and life satisfaction will surely increase.

As you try to respond to problems in a disarming and effective way, remember that most people mean well. It's just that they make lots of mistakes and misunderstand much of what they see (just like you and me). Try to get on "their side of the fence," and try to stay there while you express your thoughts and feelings. Most people will respond well. Furthermore, if a person responds poorly, you can learn a lot about that person from her reaction.

Most important, remember that you don't need to "come out on top" in order to "win." Choosing to be assertive instead of aggressive or passive is, in itself, a major victory.

BUILDING ALLIES AND LETTING GO

If we learn to influence the people around us in a nonaggressive fashion, we can decrease the pressure that supports diet/weight obsession and eating disorders by undermining fattism, the objectification of human beings, the effectiveness of advertisements, films, and other media that encourage diet/weight conflict, myths about diet and weight control, pressure to worry about diet and weight, and desires and efforts to conform to harmful aesthetic ideals.

As you begin to do this, however, beware of pouring too much of your energy into others. Remember that as much as you would like to change the world, you also want to *let go* of your preoccupation. This requires a lot of time and energy. The primary goal of educating relatives and friends is to create a haven of sorts—to ensure that the people closest to you, at least, won't be destructive influences. Hopefully, you can build a few dedicated allies.

As you gain freedom from your preoccupation, it will become easier to be exposed to negative influences without being harmed. While you are still immersed in your preoccupation, however, your tolerance may be very low. If you are unable to direct destructive conversations in a different direction, you may need to walk away. You may want to avoid especially fattist or sexist people, as well as those who often discuss their eating and weight. You may want to avoid media such as pornography and films that objectify people. The negative effects of such influences can be very powerful. They can stir up and intensify desires to be model thin, make you feel dissatisfied and anxious about your body, and encourage you to restrict and manipulate your diet. Ultimately, you want to be free to go anywhere and be with anyone without being upset by destructive influences. But if certain situations or people are very hurtful, remember that you can seek out different situations and different people. Avoidance is often a very appropriate choice.

In short, an endless stream of influences support the development and maintenance of diet/weight obsession. We must change this situation. Otherwise, diet/weight obsession and eating disorders will continue to flourish in epidemic proportions, and we will find it very difficult to free ourselves. We cannot hope to create an environment that undermines our preoccupation without influencing the attitudes and behavior of (at least) the significant people in our lives. Armed with knowledge and good will, we can begin a chain reaction. If we change the way our friends and relatives think about the central issues surrounding diet and weight, perhaps each of them will have an effect on the views of someone they know, and so on. . . . So many people are severely preoccupied with diet and weight! If as few as 5 or 10 percent of us enlighten our friends and relatives, we will soon see a blossoming social movement toward a healthier and saner view of our bodies, our eating, and ourselves.

PERSONAL QUESTIONS:
EXPLORING YOUR PRESENT ENVIRONMENT AND NEEDS

1. Make a list of the people who are very important to you. Next to each name, describe the ways in which that person *supports* your struggle for *freedom* from the diet/weight obsession.

PEOPLE	THEIR SUPPORTIVE BEHAVIOR/ATTITUDES

2. Make another list of the people who are very important to you. Next to each name, describe the ways in which that person encourages your diet/weight obsession.

PEOPLE	THEIR DESTRUCTIVE BEHAVIOR/ATTITUDES

3. What negative influences, if any, demand your immediate attention? For instance, is there a particular person who has an especially negative effect on the way you feel about your body, eating, etc.? If so, write a script in which you use "disarming and effective" communication to make him/her aware of the problem. Try to make it as realistic as possible, but give it a satisfying and peaceful ending!

4. Look at the list of negative influences in the chart below. For each one, indicate its degree of harm (for you) by circling N (for "none"), S (for "some"), or T (for "tremendous"). In the right-hand column, indicate where you would like to decrease the negative influence by circling N (for "nowhere"), I (for "my immediate environment"), or E (for "everywhere: my immediate environment and in general").

NEGATIVE INFLUENCES	DEGREE OF HARM	WHERE TO DECREASE
	None/Some/Tremendous	Nowhere/ Immediate Environment/ Everywhere
fattism in media	N S T	N I E
fattism expressed by people	N S T	N I E
objectification in media	N S T	N I E
objectification by people	N S T	N I E
weight-loss propaganda (media)	N S T	N I E
weight-loss propaganda (people)	N S T	N I E
direct pressure to worry about diet and weight	N S T	N I E

5. How can you more fully benefit from the people in your life who are supportive of your steps forward?

6. Can you create a more supportive environment for yourself by avoiding certain activities or people? If so, what or who are they?

Expressing Our Rights and Needs

7. When was the last time you noticed someone saying or doing something that supported diet/weight obsession? What did the person do or say?

8. How did you react? How did you feel about the way you reacted? If you were dissatisfied, how would you have liked to react?

9. Does it help you to recognize influences that support diet/weight obsession as such? Why or why not?

10. Do you usually stand up for your own needs? If not, why not? Do you feel that you deserve to be heard? Why or why not?

11. Do you usually *ask* for what you want (when the requests are reasonable)?

- If not, how can you begin to do so?

- What resources do you have to help you?

- What will your challenges be?

- What steps must you take to learn to make reasonable requests on a regular basis?

12.   If you could ask *and receive* any realistic favor or assistance from an important person in your life right now, what would it be? Can you ask for it now? Why or why not?

13.   Are there particular kinds of situations in which you often need to assert yourself but don't? If so, describe the situations. Why it is difficult for you to assert yourself in those situations?

14.   Do you think you could benefit by reading an instructive book (or taking a course) on assertiveness? If so, when can you begin?

15. Before going on to Chapter 8, skip ahead to Chapter 10. Read the chapter, and when you get to "Assessing Your Present Behavior," assess *your own* behavior. This will help you determine what you need to work on in order to become a good example to others.

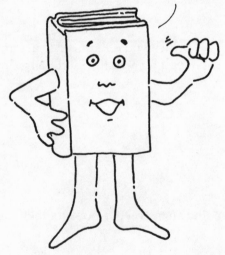

8

NUTRITIONAL GUIDELINES AND SPONTANEITY: DEVELOPING A HEALTHY LIFE-STYLE

Up until now I have said very little about one of the central (and most easily recognized) causes of diet/weight conflict: the fact that although we are pressured to be thin, we are also encouraged to "live fat." On the one hand, we are constantly told to go on weight-loss diets, join health clubs, exercise, and lose weight. At the same time, we are encouraged to "go with the flow" of American life—eat "normal" foods, participate in social events that include drinking and eating, and work at a sedentary job. If we go with this flow, then our diets will tend to be high in sugar and fat and low in fiber, and we will tend to be very sedentary. Thus we will embrace a life-style that promotes relatively high setpoints.

The cult surrounding diets, diet food, exercise programs, etc., actually attests to these contradictory pressures. We want to live

"normally" *and* be thin. Consequently, we look for quick weight-loss schemes and nonnutritional sugar and fat substitutes to solve our dilemma. We want to follow a certain program, lose weight, and then return to our normal way of life without regaining weight. Given all the common assumptions about the energy balance, this is not an unreasonable thing to expect. But because the assumptions are faulty (see Chapter 2), it doesn't work.

The goal of this book is to help you attain freedom from diet/weight conflict. Realize, however, that even within that freedom you will be pressured to accept a "normal" life-style (which is less than ideal for your health), and even within that freedom you will have to decide what you want to eat and how much you want to exercise. The purpose of this chapter is to help you recognize the tremendous life-style pressures you will have to sort out in order to make those choices. Through the questions and exercises, you can then begin to envision *your* ideal life-style.

THE AMERICAN FOOD INDUSTRY

The food industry and the media have a strong effect on what we eat. We *can* restrict our diets to fresh fruits, vegetables, legumes, and whole grains; however, we are encouraged to eat all kinds of "normal" prepared foods. What is the content of many of the foods we are encouraged to eat? Most prepared foods* contain processed grains, simple sugars,† and/or a lot of fat.

Sugar is an especially interesting example. Since the end of World War II, Americans have been eating more and more sugar. We are using less sugar in our homes, which creates the illusion that we are eating less sugar; however, the food industry is using *more* sugar.[1] Consequently, a person who never adds sugar to anything and avoids all obvious sweets nonetheless eats sugar. Food producers add some form of simple sugar to most beverages, breads, cereals, crackers, canned foods, flavored yogurt, fast-food hamburgers, and hundreds of other common foods.

We can read labels to see if sugar is listed, but first we must learn all the different names for simple sugars. They include corn syrup, sucrose, glucose, dextrose, maltose, lactose, fructose, honey, and molasses. Furthermore, labels do not list amounts, so they provide only a vague idea of how much sugar we eat.

How many people know that most colas contain approximately *nine teaspoons* of sugar per twelve-ounce serving? How many parents realize that some of the cereals they buy for their children are over 60 percent sugar? Most Americans unknowingly eat an enormous amount of sugar.

One of the reasons why food producers are adding more and more sugar to prepared foods is that people like the taste and immediate physical lift it provides. Furthermore, tastes are to some extent determined by conditioning: we expect bread or orange juice to be extra sweet if it has always tasted that way. Early conditioning creates popular demand in a vicious cycle. A large proportion of foods contain added sugar (starting with baby foods); therefore, people are conditioned to expect their foods to be sweet and may become "addicted" to sugar.[2] Thus the demand for sweet foods is high, and in some instances increasing sugar content may increase sales. In response, the food industry adds more and more sugar to more and more foods, and more people become conditioned to expect foods to be sweet . . . and so on.

Advertisements also affect the American diet. Although children and uneducated

---

* All foods that contain many different ingredients are "prepared foods." This category includes a large proportion of what most people buy: bread, crackers, soup, cereals, soda, most canned foods, most frozen foods, etc.

† Simple sugars include all mono- and disaccharides (we consume primarily the latter) in forms such as white sugar, honey, syrups, and molasses. These are different from polysaccharides, otherwise known as complex carbohydrates or starches. This distinction is important because all simple sugars are metabolized very quickly and provide a rush of energy and satisfaction, swiftly followed by a complete lack of energy and renewed hunger. Complex carbohydrates, on the other hand, are metabolized more gradually, and thus provide less concentrated energy for a much longer period of time.

adults may be the most susceptible, even a health-conscious adult can be misled by advertising unless she reads labels carefully and is armed with knowledge about foods and nutrition.

As consumers have become more concerned about their diets, manufacturers have made liberal use of catchwords and phrases such as "100 percent natural," "nothing artificial," "sugar free," "fortified," and "diet." These terms are too loosely defined to be helpful to us. They are misleading marketing devices that are successfully used to increase sales.[3] For instance, many products labeled "no sugar added" or "sugarless" contain some form of sugar. In these products the "no sugar" label really means no white table sugar or brown sugar. This is very misleading because *all* simple sugars, including those in honey, molasses, and maple syrup, have the same (negative) effect on our bodies.[4]

Breads provide another important example of misleading labeling. Health-conscious consumers are looking for whole grain breads and trying to avoid breads made of processed (white) flour. In response, many manufacturers have used names like "wheat bread" to increase sales of white bread. Some even use molasses or coloring to make white bread look like whole wheat bread! Consequently, many consumers think they are eating whole wheat bread when actually eating white bread. (To avoid this trap, look for labels that say "100% *Whole* Wheat," or read the ingredient list. If "wheat flour" or "enriched flour" is listed, then it isn't whole wheat.)

Not all slogans and commercials are deceptive. However, all commercials attempt to convince consumers to buy products. The $7–$9 billion devoted to food advertising every year (not including alcoholic beverages) attests to their effectiveness. If advertising was not effective, it would not account for 3 to 3.7 cents of every dollar Americans spend on food at home.[5] Thus much of the American diet is determined by catchy advertising rather than by careful decisions based on content, quality, and taste.

In order to avoid a "normal" diet that is high in fat, sugar, and processed grains, we could limit our intake to unprepared foods and carefully selected prepared foods. However, even these guidelines would not protect us from a diet high in fat. Many unprepared foods often considered "healthy" or "diet" foods are actually very high in fat. For instance, many people think of red meat as a "protein food." It would be equally appropriate to think of it as a "fat food." A "choice" (broiled) sirloin steak, for instance, contains 34–45 percent fat by weight. Nuts are another so-called "protein food." Most varieties are over 50 percent fat by weight.

In short, strong influences such as food industry policies, advertising, and a lack of nutritional education lead most Americans to eat lots of sugar, fat, and refined carbohydrates. Perhaps even more important, the proliferation of restaurants, the overwhelming quantity of food-related advertising, and the way in which many social and business events revolve around eating and drinking all lead to continual food consciousness and food availability. Thus we are surrounded by opposing messages: "Eat here!" "Try food X!" "Eat delicious food Y!"; and "Be thin!" "Eat less!" "Eat the right foods!" "Go on diet X, Y, or Z!" It's little wonder that so many of us suffer from conflicting desires and diet/weight obsession.

EXERCISE AND THE "AMERICAN WAY OF LIFE"

Since the beginning of the industrial revolution, we have rapidly and systematically decreased the amount of physical exertion required for survival by replacing human power with machine power. The number of jobs that involve physical exertion are at an all-time low because machines now do much of the work that used to require physical labor. In addition, we have drastically decreased the amount of human energy needed to move from place to place with cars, planes, buses, subways, elevators, escalators, and moving sidewalks. We have further decreased the amount of energy needed in everyday life with vacuum cleaners, washing machines, dishwashers, blenders, food processors, snowblowers, snowplows, and other machines and gadgets.

Now that we have made it possible to be sedentary, we find it difficult to be otherwise. Most of us must work at sedentary jobs for forty hours a week (or more), and we are likely to have further responsibilities that take time: maintaining our households, taking care of children, cooking. . . . Furthermore, if we don't happen to enjoy running or doing calisthenics, we may need to spend money for club memberships, class fees, and equipment in order to enjoy exercise. In our culture, exercise has become a luxury that requires time *and* money. Many basic demands (for survival) conspire against our desire and need for exercise.

The media often imply that exercise is a simple matter of personal choice. In a sense, this is true. Most of us could make regular exercise a priority. However, this assumption ignores the fact that, as in the case of our eating habits, we are surrounded by contradictory influences. We are told that we should exercise regularly; however, we are socialized to have a sedentary life-style.

SPONTANEOUS AND HEALTHY LIVING

Throughout this book I have suggested that you can eat spontaneously, stop being obsessed with your body, exercise for pleasure and fitness, focus on more important matters, and thus attain freedom from your diet/weight obsession. I still maintain that this is so. But what then? What will you be eating, and how will you be living? Will you be a junk food junkie? Will you be sedentary? Will you be unhealthy and unfit? Obviously, *you* will determine the answers to these questions for yourself. I have been teaching you to attain freedom from your preoccupation, *not* to relinquish responsibility for your own choices.

Everyone must choose her own life-style: those who have never suffered from a diet/weight obsession, those who suffer from a diet/weight obsession, *and* those who have freed themselves from a diet/weight obsession. The flow of life in this society promotes an unhealthy diet and a lack of exercise; however, you can choose to go with the flow or you can choose to do something different. One of the joys of being free from diet/weight conflict is that within a state of freedom it is much easier (and much more pleasurable) to choose a healthy life-style despite cultural pressure to do otherwise. And a common (though not universal) benefit of having been preoccupied with diet and weight is some knowledge about food content and nutrition. You may be in a better position to make healthy food-related decisions than most of the people who have never been preoccupied with diet and weight.

When you are free from your preoccupation, you will not be free from the conflict between your desire to be healthy and the cultural pressures that promote an unhealthy life-style. You will still be surrounded by fast food chains, ice cream trucks, soda machines, and candy machines, and you will still be living in a society that encourages you to work a lot but exercise very little. However, you will be able to make your choices in freedom. You can choose whatever life-style feels best to you. You can choose a life-style that may not promote extreme slenderness, but instead promotes your health and well-being.

What is all this talk about "choosing" eating habits? What happended to "spontaneous eating?" Nothing happened to it. I still recommend that you relearn to eat in a spontaneous way. However, I've never met anyone who felt a strong craving along with every hunger pang. Most of the time your body will be less specific about its needs, and you will have to decide what to eat. You can make your eating decisions partly based on nutritional considerations, yet eat in a spontaneous way. Even spontaneous eaters make choices when they walk into a grocery store and shop for food. Even spontaneous eaters tend to eat some things very often and other things less often or not at all. You, too, will have to decide what to eat no matter how spontaneous your eating becomes.

At first, chronic dieters tend to feel that if they aren't eating a lot of junky food, then they couldn't really be eating spontaneously. They don't believe that they could really be eating whatever they want whenever they want. This is a natural assumption given that they are emerging from chronic attempts to deprive themselves. They have assumed that they always want disallowed food. So, if they are not always eating what used to be disallowed, they feel as though they couldn't possibly be eating what they want.

This is not the case. I eat spontaneously, but I *also* eat in a very healthy way. As you work toward spontaneous eating and freedom from your preoccupation, try to eat in a joyful, pleasurable, and satisfying way. However, remember to allow yourself to make healthy choices. Healthy eating, too, can be joyful, pleasurable, satisfying, and spontaneous.

How would you most *like* to eat? While fully immersed in a diet/weight obsession and the pursuit of slenderness, the answer was clear: "whatever way it takes to become and remain thin." Consequently, you lacked the freedom to choose a comfortable life-style that would support your health and happiness. You were too obsessed, too self-destructive, too determined to fight with your body . . . perhaps you still are. But what if you were completely free from diet/weight conflict and the pursuit of slenderness? *Then* how would you like to be eating?

You may benefit from envisioning the way you would like to eat—envisioning spontaneous, flexible eating that is nutritionally sound. You may not want to develop this vision right away. You may need to spend a long while just "feeling yourself out"—eating according to every whim, and concentrating on what you feel and what you really want. Don't feel that you have to develop a new vision right away. However, many people find it helpful to create a vision of ideal eating, even before they have attained the basis of freedom needed to realize that vision.

What nutritional guidelines should you use to develop this vision? Different "experts" have different ideas about what is healthy. If you are one of the many chronic dieters, anorexics, or bulimics who have read every book on nutrition and weight loss with obsessive interest, then you are in the same position I am. You know a lot about what everyone and his nephew thinks on the subject, and you are free to believe whatever or whomever you like.

If, on the other hand, you have *not* experienced this particular obsession, you may know little more than a few popular myths about nutrition. In this case, you may want to discard the clearly faulty information and replace it with some useful current ideas.

My workshop participants always want to know what choices I've made. They want to know what I eat and how much I exercise. I usually answer their questions, but I make it clear that there is no such thing as "*the* way" to eat and live. It's sensible to base your choices on nutritional and health concerns; however, you need to remember that as soon as you embrace a certain diet as "the solution" to your problem, you run the risk of once again getting caught up in potentially harmful "shoulds," "should nots," and dieters' mind-set.

For this reason, I originally omitted nutritional information from my workshops and this book. I did not want to fall into the trap of providing yet another "diet." However, it has since come to my attention that many people who suffer from diet/weight conflict struggle with "shoulds" and "should nots" that would *not* promote good health and high energy levels (or a lower setpoint) even if followed. Furthermore, many sufferers do not know how to fill their cupboards with delicious, healthy foods, or how to prepare delicious, healthy meals.

I had to ask myself: "Would I have attained this joyous state of freedom had I not known, at least in theory, how to eat *well?*" Perhaps not. At the very least, I would not have eaten as much nourishing food, would not have felt as energetic, healthy, or happy, and, therefore, would not have been as motivated to keep working toward real freedom.

If you are at a point where you need to abandon all prescriptions regarding your eating, then stop right here and skip ahead to Chapter 9. For instance, if you already know a lot about nutrition and need, first and foremost, to break free from dieters' mind-set, then you should probably skip this section. However, if you know little about nutrition and feel that a vision of healthy eating would be helpful, then read on.

DIETERS' MYTHS

First, try to let go of any nutritional *myths* that may be affecting your eating in a negative way. The most popular of these myths is that starchy foods like bread, pasta, potatoes, and rice (often called "complex carbohydrates") are fattening and low in nutritional value. This is simply untrue.

Starchy foods are actually less fattening than many of the so-called diet foods, such as meat and cottage cheese. This is because starchy foods are virtually fat free, and fats of all kinds tend to raise setpoint, *unlike* starch. Furthermore, our bodies "waste" more of the calories derived from complex carbohydrates than those derived from protein. Jane Brody, a widely respected nutritionist and author, cites two reasons for this waste: (a) carbohydrates cause more calories to be burned up as heat (which helps you feel warm); (b) up to a third of complex carbohydrate calories are not digested, but are excreted unabsorbed.[6] Thus, as far as your body is concerned, they "don't count."

When people do not eat enough complex carbohydrates, they usually feel tired and listless. Not only is this a very unpleasant side effect of low-carbohydrate diets, it tends to lead to a decrease in physical movement, which in turn translates into lower caloric needs. A lack of complex carbohydrates also causes carbohydrate cravings, which in turn can lead to bingeing. In short, starchy foods are not "fattening." In fact, the opposite seems to be true: when a dieter eats more starchy foods, her weight often decreases.[7]

As for nutritional value, starchy foods are very nutritious provided they are not ruined through processing. For instance, wheat is very nutritious unless twenty-six nutrients are "milled out" in order to make *white* flour.[8] Enriched white flour has had four of these nutrients put back, but fiber, among other good things, is left out. This is too bad, since fiber is essential to good health but sadly lacking in the typical highly processed American diet. In short, starchy foods are an essential part of healthy eating. If you eat whole grain bread, whole wheat pasta, potatoes, brown rice, and other grains that have not been processed, these foods will be nutritious as well as delicious and satisfying.

Another popular myth is that meat is a healthy "diet food." Over and over I see people ordering two hamburgers or hot dogs without the rolls, the assumption being that it's "better for you" to eat more protein and less starch. The truth is that meat, especially red meat, is very high in saturated fat, and diets high in saturated fat have been linked to numerous health problems in addition to raising setpoint weight. More frightening still are the health problems that may arise as a result of the chemicals, hormones, and antibiotics in today's meats (except in "organic meat").[9] In short, the idea that meat is a healthy "diet food" is simply wrong.

The idea that protein is some kind of "wonder" nutrient, of which we can't get enough, is also a myth. Many people focus on trying to eat a lot of protein, not realizing that their protein needs are very easily met. For instance, a woman who weighs 138 pounds has an RDA (recommended daily allowance) of approximately 50 grams of protein, assuming she is neither pregnant nor breast-feeding. She could easily meet this RDA by eating one cup of oatmeal (11 grams of protein), one cup of milk (8 grams), one tuna fish sandwich (21 grams), and one cup of pea soup (11 grams). Furthermore, scientists purposely set the RDA for protein 30 percent *above* most people's requirements, so most women of 138 pounds could meet their actual protein need even more easily than the above example demonstrates.

Even vegetarians can meet their protein needs without too much effort. However, they must be aware that vegetable proteins are not nutritionally complete and must therefore be combined in specific ways in order to create complete, usable protein. To accomplish this, you can:

- combine legumes (dried peas and beans or peanuts) with grains.

- combine legumes with nuts and seeds.

- combine eggs or dairy products with any vegetable protein.[10]

In short, we don't need to eat an enormous amount of protein. In fact, most Americans eat far more protein than they need, at the expense of eating too much fat and not enough complex carbohydrates.

Last, but not least, is the myth that nonnutritive sweeteners aid in weight control. Studies have demonstrated that replacing sugar with nonnutritive sweeteners does not lower weight. In fact, preliminary evidence indicates that nonnutritive sweeteners may elevate setpoint weight just like sugar.[11] If this is so, then dieters who drink large quantities of diet soda are doing themselves a great disservice. Not only are they ingesting many potentially harmful chemicals, they are probably boosting their setpoint weights, the opposite of their intention.

THE BASICS OF HEALTHY EATING

Our understanding of what constitutes "healthy eating" is forever changing. In the 1930s and 1940s, for instance, nutritionists were primarily concerned with preventing nutrient *deficiency* and resulting health problems such as pellagra and rickets. Today, on the other hand, nutritionists are more concerned with preventing the *overconsumption* of fats, salt, and refined sugars, which seems to increase the chances of developing hypertension, heart disease, and stroke.

Over time, we see a lot of "experts" come and go. Most of them offer slight variations on current or past nutritional themes, while only a few offer new and radical ideas, many of which prove to be unhealthy fads in the final analysis. I am going to focus on mainstream ideas that are, at present, in favor with most nutritionists, because (a) I believe that these ideas have been the best supported by scientific evidence, and (b) my own experience has confirmed that nutritionists' current conception of healthy eating leads to feeling good and energetic.

Nutritionists agree that most Americans need to (a) eat a variety of foods, (b) avoid too much fat, saturated fat, and cholesterol, (c) eat foods with adequate starch and fiber, (d) avoid too much sugar, (e) avoid too much sodium (i.e., salt), and (f) drink alcohol, if at all, in moderation. The consensus is that 12 percent of our daily calories should be derived from protein, between 10 and 30 percent from fat, and between 58 and 78 percent from carbohydrates. Most nutritionists suggest a compromise on the percentage of fat. For instance, Bonnie Liebman and the authors of "Nutrition Action" recommend a compromise of 20–25 percent of calories from fat.[12]

This high-carbohydrate way of eating feels *wonderful*. It requires that we eat lots of substantial, delicious, filling, energy-giving food! Chronic dieters tend to be especially pleased by this way of eating because they have been suffering from the side effects of low-carbohydrate intake, which can include low energy levels, carbohydrate cravings, hunger (sometimes even after meals), irritability, and being oversensitive to cold.

If you decide to try high-carbohydrate eating, there is no need to do so for "weight loss," even though it may lead to some. Instead, aim for feeling more energetic, for staying warm where you used to feel cold, for a happier mood, for feeling more satisfied during and after meals, for the enjoyment of pasta, potatoes, breads, rice, and other wonderful grains, and for the good health and longevity this nutritious eating is likely to engender. By focusing on these benefits rather than on lowering setpoint, you can more easily avoid the trap of letting healthy eating become another "diet."

How can you go about switching to the recommended distribution of protein, fat, and carbohydrates outlined above? Many books and leaflets are available to teach you how to play the numbers game of figuring out your current distribution. Or, if you prefer, you can go to a local nutritionist and pay her to analyze your current diet and help you identify advisable changes. My own recommendation is: don't bother with the numbers. Playing the numbers game usually encourages dieters' mind-set and diet/weight preoccupation, particularly if you already suffer from these problems. Even if you begin to do it with health considerations in mind, the numbers tend to suck you into a dieter's way of thinking.

Instead, I recommend that you begin by buying cookbooks that can teach you to cook healthy, delicious meals, and use their recipes on a regular basis. This alone can improve the quality of your diet enormously with a minimum of effort and *without feeling deprived*.

The best cookbooks of this nature that I've found are listed in the "Recommended Reading" section of Resources (p. 240). If you can't afford to buy more than one, buy the *Good Food Book* by Jane Brody. This book alone can serve the purpose admirably for many years before you could feel you'd "tried it all" and needed to branch out. However, if you are a chronic dieter, bulimic, or anorexic, I suggest that you do *not* read the nutrition section at the beginning. Just use the recipes. Brody's nutritional information is current and accurate; however, her writing sometimes incorporates fattist attitudes that are less than helpful to people who are obsessed with, or upset by, their weight and eating.

We have a tremendous variety of foods at our disposal. Food varies a lot, of course, in terms of nutritional quality. Let me share with you my own way of thinking about and dealing with different kinds of food. This isn't *the way* of thinking and eating; it's just my way. I find it very pleasant and spontaneous, yet healthy. Perhaps you will want to borrow from it as you develop *your way* of eating.

I think of my eating in terms of "habitual eating," "additional eating," and "recreational eating." The habitual eating refers to the foods and meals I eat on a habitual basis. These are foods of excellent nutritional quality in that they all provide necessary nutrients with a minimum of fat, sugar, salt, or processed grain. I keep these staples in stock at home, and automatically focus my eating around them.

"Additional eating" refers to foods that I also eat fairly often, but that I do not think of as habitual foods because they are high in fat, sugar, salt, or processed grain relative to my staple foods. The additional eating is a very significant part, but doesn't represent the *bulk*, of my food intake. In other words, I eat the additional foods less frequently or in smaller amounts than the habitual foods.

"Recreational eating" is just that: purely recreational. I enjoy all of my eating, but *most* of it serves *two* purposes: (a) satisfying nutritional needs and (b) giving me pleasure. Recreational eating, on the other hand, serves only the latter purpose. Therefore, it is for the fulfillment of cravings and "fun times" or special events. And if I am not going to *fully enjoy* eating a recreational food for some reason, then I skip it, since it serves no purpose other than enjoyment. For instance, if I am in a hurry or am already full, then I wait for a better time. When I do eat recreationally, I enjoy it to the fullest without guilt or anxiety. That way I derive the greatest possible enjoyment and satisfaction, which is the whole point of eating these foods.

Another important aspect of my eating is that I virtually *never* eat certain foods, because (a) I actively dislike the taste or texture of them, or (b) I don't like them enough to choose them over other nutritionally equivalent, but in my opinion much tastier, foods, or (c) equally delicious but nutritionally superior alternatives are available. Some of the foods that fall into one of these three categories *for me* include white bread, whole milk, avocado (except in guacamole—yum), peanut butter, canned fruit, sweet breakfast cereals, potato chips, french fries, soda, most fried food, and red meat.

In other words, these are foods I don't eat because I prefer the taste of many other foods with the same or better nutritional quality. But I'm not rigid about it. If there are no other options owing to circumstances beyond my control, then I eat the available food rather than go hungry. If I have a choice, as I usually do, then I choose what I like most.

This seems very basic and obvious. However, it is a useful point because I used to eat all sorts of things I didn't like very much. I was in the habit of doing so, first because I had to eat whatever my mother served me as a child, and second because I was limited to what was offered in a cafeteria for a few years after that. I find that a lot of people have developed the same habit: eating things they don't like all that much, even if the nutritional quality is only mediocre, or worse. This is a habit well worth changing.

Of course, you have to decide on *your own* likes and dislikes. I only supplied my "yucko list" to serve as an example. If you are already skipping the foods you find only marginally enjoyable, great. But if you're not, you might like to determine which ones are only fair in nutritional quality or downright unhealthy, and skip them to make room for other foods you like better.

The following chart lists a wide variety of foods (not just the ones I happen to like) by type: (1) grains, beans, and nuts; (2) fruits and vegetables; (3) milk products; (4) poultry, fish, meat, and eggs; and (5) miscellaneous. Within each type, the foods are classified as habitual, additional, or recreational based upon their nutritional quality. The habitual foods are of excellent quality, the additional foods are of reasonable but lesser quality (because of fat, sugar, processed grain, or salt content), and the recreational foods are of relatively poor nutritional quality.

Note that if you want your food energy to be derived approximately 12 percent from protein, 20–25 percent from fat, and 63–68 percent from carbohydrates, you will want to eat the bulk of your food from categories 1 and 2 (grains, beans, vegetables, and fruits), and smaller amounts from categories 3 and 4 (milk and animal products). Likewise, you will want the bulk of your food to come under the "habitual" category, less from "additional," and still less from "recreational."

I try to eat a very wide variety of foods. I love eating and I love discovering new foods. Go into a large supermarket and walk up and down the aisles looking for food you don't recognize or have never tried. You'll be amazed by how much food is unfamiliar. Try some new grains; try some new vegetables; try a new variety of fish. You may be happily surprised by all the delicious foods you have been missing.

Most people who struggle with diet and weight get into a very repetitive pattern of eating. We find ourselves eating a few "safe" and familiar foods over and over. If this pattern becomes too restricted, it can lead to poor nutrition because it is only by eating a *variety* of foods that we get all the vitamins, minerals, complex carbohydrates, fat, and protein we need. Today I find that if I follow my instincts and cravings, then, in general, I end up eating in a well-balanced way. However, when first breaking out of a restricted eating pattern, a few guidelines can be helpful.

The Center for Science in the Public Interest recommends that we try to eat four *or more* servings from the beans, grains, and nuts category, four *or more* servings from fruits and vegetables, two servings from milk products, and two servings from the poultry, fish, meat, and eggs category (vegetarians can substitute from the other groups).[13] If, in addition, you strive for variety *within* each category, you can be certain of eating a variety of foods as recommended by most nutritionists. (For example, from the fruits and vegetables category, eat spinach, carrots, an orange, and a banana rather than four servings of a single fruit or vegetable.)

I did not *consciously* develop my way of thinking about food and eating. Instead, it gradually evolved out of two basic goals: (a) to eat spontaneously and (b) to eat healthily. My eating reflects the above nutritional concepts; however, I ate this way for years without consciously categorizing foods and without verbalizing any of the underlying principles.

It is also important to understand that I

HABITUAL STAPLE FOODS	ADDITIONAL FOODS	RECREATIONAL FOODS

1. Grains, Beans, and Nuts

HABITUAL STAPLE FOODS	ADDITIONAL FOODS	RECREATIONAL FOODS
Brown rice	White rice	Croissants
Whole grain bread	White bread	Doughnuts
Whole wheat pasta	Refined pasta	Stuffing (traditional)
Whole grain, unsweetened cereals	Refined, unsweetened cereals	Presweetened cereals
Dried beans and peas	Granola cereals	Cakes
Whole grain pancakes	Refried beans	Pastries
Whole wheat matzoh	Pancakes with syrup	Waffles with syrup
Whole grain flatbread or Wasa	Matzoh	Cookies
Popcorn, air-popped or with minimal oil and salt	Low-fat crackers	Regular crackers
Tofu	Regular popcorn with butter and salt	
Bulgur	Cornbread	
Lentils	Flour tortillas	
Oatmeal	Macaroni and cheese	
Sprouts	Nuts and seeds	
Corn (on the cob)	Peanut butter	
Whole wheat bagels	Pizza	
	Bagels	
	Couscous	

2. Fruits and Vegetables

HABITUAL STAPLE FOODS	ADDITIONAL FOODS	RECREATIONAL FOODS
All vegetables except those listed elsewhere	Avocado	Coconut
All fruits except those listed elsewhere	Coleslaw	Pickles
Unsweetened applesauce	Dried fruit	
Potatoes	Fruit canned in syrup	
Unsweetened fruit juices	Sweetened applesauce	
Vegetable juices	Potatoes au gratin	Potato chips
	Sweetened fruit juices	French fries
	Cranberry sauce	

continued

HABITUAL STAPLE FOODS	ADDITIONAL FOODS	RECREATIONAL FOODS
	3. Milk Products	
Skim or 1% low-fat milk	2% low-fat milk	Half & Half
Low-fat yogurt, plain	Low-fat yogurt,	Cream
Low-fat cottage cheese	sweetened	Ice cream
Skim milk cheeses	Whole milk cottage	Ice milk
	cheese	Cream cheese
	Part-skim cheeses	Frozen yogurt
	Processed and hard	Cheesecake
	cheeses*	Sour Cream
	Whole milk	

	4. Poultry, Fish, Meat, and Eggs	
Bass	Fried fish	Bacon
Cod	Herring	Beef liver, fried
Flounder	Mackerel	Bologna
Gefilte fish	Salmon (and lox)	Corned beef
Haddock	Sardines	Ground beef
Halibut		Ham
Perch		Hot dogs
Pollock		Liverwurst
Rockfish		Salami
Sole		Sausage
Trout		Spare ribs
Tuna (in water)	Tuna (in oil)	Commercial fried
Shellfish	Fried chicken in	chicken
Shrimp	vegetable oil	Untrimmed red meats
Swordfish	Lean red meats	Pig's feet
Chicken or turkey,	Eggs (or yolks)	
boiled, broiled, baked,		
or roasted		
Egg whites		
Sushi		

continued

* One could argue for putting hard cheeses under "recreational" because of high saturated fat content. Consider them to be halfway between the two categories.

Nutritional Guidelines and Spontaneity: Developing a Healthy Life-Style

HABITUAL STAPLE FOODS	ADDITIONAL FOODS	RECREATIONAL FOODS
	5. Miscellaneous	
Water	Herbal tea	Sodas
Grain beverages:	Regular tea	Diet sodas
Postum, Cafix	Decaffeinated coffee	Alcoholic beverages
Mustard	Regular coffee	Candy
Oil-free salad dressings:	Reduced-fat salad	Regular salad dressings
Yogurt-based	dressings	Regular mayonnaise
dressings	Reduced-fat mayonnaise	"Health food bars"
Lemon juice with		(candy)
spices		Deep-fried foods
Vinegar with spices	Commercial soups	Sugar, syrup, etc.
Rice-based dressings		
Homemade soups (low	Margarine (small	Butter
salt)	amounts)	
Vegetable oil for cooking		
(small amounts)		

take a rather relaxed approach to all of the above in order to preserve my spontaneity and guard against dieters' mind-set. I try to eat in a healthy way each day, but I don't keep track of how much of my food is from the various categories, or how much food I'm eating. I just eat spontaneously with the quiet intention and habit of eating *mostly* healthy foods.

This relaxed approach has allowed my "tastes" to follow all sorts of trends and preferences. Sometimes I develop a passion for a certain food I rarely used to eat and find myself having it on a regular basis. If it's one of my staple foods, then the "trend" is hardly noticeable and certainly of no concern. If it's an additional or recreational food, then I enjoy it (in moderation) nonetheless.

Eventually, I always move on to other favorites, so I don't let the less healthy trends bother me.

For instance, earlier this year I was temporarily in love with bagels with ricotta cheese (only the whole milk variety tasted good to me). It became a daily snack. I don't think of these as staple foods, because of their respective refined grain and fat content. But I nonetheless ate them regularly and didn't worry about it. Now I'm sick of them, so I'm back to eating bagels and ricotta much less often, which is fine.

I have put my way of thinking about food and eating into words here because I hope that it will help you to develop *your own* way of eating without forfeiting spontaneity or good nutrition. Once again, let me caution you: I am not trying to overshadow you with more dos and don'ts. Instead, I have tried to offer a few basics of good nutrition in a way that should not encourage dieters' mind-set or diet/weight conflict.

As you develop your own vision of "ideal" eating, try to give yourself the space to *evolve into* eating the way you envision. It is very difficult, and tends to feel like another diet, if you try to change the way you eat in a drastic way, all at once. This tends to promote temporary rather than lasting change, and temporary change can be worse than no change at all, since it will feel like another failure.

On the other hand, I guarantee that as long as you train yourself to eat whatever *amount* of food you want and never allow yourself to go hungry, healthy eating will be much easier to achieve than following any limited or low-calorie diet. This is because you will not be struggling against your hunger signals. Instead, you will be able to eat in harmony with your body's needs and will therefore feel comfortable, sated, and energetic.

Give yourself plenty of time. If you don't care for many of the foods that fall into the habitual category, give yourself the time and opportunity to develop a taste for some of those foods. Most people come to prefer almost anything that they eat on a regular basis. For instance, I used to dislike whole wheat bread because I was brought up on white bread. However, having gradually replaced white bread with whole wheat, I find that I don't like white bread anymore: it seems tasteless and mushy now. The same thing occurred with milk: I used to like whole milk, now I prefer skim milk. Thus what we like is, to a large extent, a matter of what is familiar and "normal" to us. If you would like to do so, you can *gradually* change what you like. If you don't want to develop these changes in taste, then don't. This, too, is a completely reasonable choice. Only you can discover what works and feels best for you.

ABOUT WATER

Many people have asked me how much water they should drink. Experts offer a wide variety of opinions, from recommending that you virtually drown yourself in it to strictly limiting liquid of all kinds. In my opinion, you should drink water whenever thirsty, but first *be sure that you know how to recognize thirst!*

It is very easy to miss the feeling of thirst or mistake it for hunger. Those who have been tuning out their hunger signals in attempts to lose weight are especially likely to be out of touch with thirst. Jane Brody says that anyone, even those in touch with their thirst, can stop feeling thirsty before drinking enough. She recommends, therefore, that you continue drinking beyond the point of quenching thirst. It is better, she believes, to err on the side of drinking too much water, since your body will simply get rid of any water it doesn't need. She recommends at least six, and preferably eight, eight-ounce glasses of liquid per day.[14]

I have had a hard time recognizing my own feelings of thirst. For years I drank so little liquid that I suffered from chronic dehydration headaches and urinary tract infections. My doctor kept telling me to drink more liquid, but it was hard to remember, and a bit unpleasant to do it, because I rarely felt thirsty except after exercising.

If you drink very little liquid, it is likely that you are out of touch with thirst. The easiest way to reconnect is to drink water even though you don't feel thirsty and see how you feel afterward. Do you feel more relaxed? Less hungry? More energetic? "Better" in some way? Any of these reactions could mean that you were thirsty without knowing it. You may even find that drinking a *little* water brings thirst to your awareness. If this works for you, simply drink small amounts of water on a regular basis to "check" for thirst.

I am much better at recognizing thirst now, but I still make a special effort to drink plenty of water. Otherwise, I tend to drink too little. When I feel hungry between meals, I drink a little water before snacking to see if I'm thirsty. I drink water after exercising and, often, after urinating. I drink water if I start to get a headache (this often wards it off). And I drink water with all of my meals despite some claims that this dilutes digestive juices and hinders digestion. (Dr. Dennis Remington says that unless you have had part of your stomach removed because of ulcers or cancer, or a hiatal hernia, there is no reason to restrict water.)[15]

I keep saying "water" rather than "liquid," because I drink mostly water. In fact, there is nothing that I drink on a *daily* basis other than water. However, this is just a personal preference. Most nutritionists feel that it is fine to drink any of the following on a regular basis: water, unsweetened fruit juice, vegetable juice, or grain beverages such as Postum or Cafix. Evidence to date indicates that moderate amounts of coffee or tea do no harm, either, except that caffeine usually backfires hours later in the form of tiredness.

Herbal teas have become very popular, and many nutritionists believe they are harmless. However, severe physical reactions to herbal teas have been reported in the medical literature, and Jane Brody recommends great caution in selecting and drinking herbal tea.[16] If you buy a new herbal tea, drink only a small amount at first to see if you have a reaction to it. If you have no reaction, then it is probably okay to drink a glass or two at a time, but it is not a good idea to drink herbal tea as if it were water—it isn't.

What about soft drinks? As you probably know, soft drinks are full of sugar and/or chemicals and, often, caffeine. It is a good idea to consider these drinks recreational fare, like cake and candy. But if you begin to drink fewer soft drinks, be sure to drink more water or other liquid! Avoiding soft drinks is very difficult *if* you forget to quench your thirst in other ways.

Many people have told me that they do not like the taste of water. If this is true for you, try some or all of the following options: (a) look for a bottled water you like; (b) put a little lemon or lime juice in your water; (c) try drinking water at different temperatures, from hot to lukewarm to cold to iced; (d) try using a water purifier if your tap water is bad; (e) try seltzer water—it has a little fizz *without* added salt, preservatives, sugar, or flavorings.

ABOUT DIETARY FAT

Virtually every nutritionist agrees that we need to avoid excessive dietary fat in order to protect our health. High fat eating has been linked to heart attack, stroke, atherosclerosis, and colon and breast cancer. Since these maladies seem well worth avoiding, foods high in fat seem well worth limiting.

But is all fat the same? No, it's more complicated than that.

The primary health hazard is high blood cholesterol. Therefore, it is helpful to limit foods that are high in cholesterol, which include eggs (250 milligrams per yolk), organ meats (370 mg/3 ounces of liver), other red meats, cheese, and whole milk (25–75 mg/serving). In addition, saturated fat *raises blood cholesterol.* Therefore, foods high in saturated fat should also be limited, including coconut oil, palm kernel oil, palm oil, chocolate, whole milk, cheese, butter, cream, beef, veal, lard, and pork.

Monounsaturated fats do not affect blood cholesterol. Foods high in these fats include avocados, fish, olive oil, almonds, peanuts, and most margarine. Polyunsaturated fats actually lower blood cholesterol. Polyunsaturated fats are found in safflower oil, sunflower oil, corn oil, soybean oil, mayonnaise, and sesame oil.

This does not mean that we should try to eat lots of polyunsaturated fats, for this, too, could be a health hazard (polyunsaturated fats have been linked to colon cancer). Instead, most nutritionists and heart experts recommend that we cut down on saturated fats and replace some saturated fats with polyunsaturated fats.

In any case, these considerations were taken into account in the preceding food chart and corresponding discussion. If you decide to try the high-carbohydrate way of eating and the *bulk* of your food comes from grains, beans, fruits, and vegetables (from under "habitual"), then your diet will not be a danger to your blood cholesterol.

ABOUT ALLERGIES

I have repeatedly received letters from people who want advice about how to develop spontaneous eating despite food allergies or food intolerances. This is a difficult problem to solve because, obviously, you cannot simply eat whatever you want whenever you want if you have negative reactions to many foods.

A food allergy is present when a certain food provokes an *immune response.* The resulting symptoms range from nausea, vomiting, or diarrhea to rashes, itching, or difficulty breathing. In very rare cases, an allergic reaction to food can even cause death. Food allergies most often involve cow's milk protein, egg whites, various kinds of nuts, and seafood. Only about 5 percent of children and less than 2 percent of adults have food allergies.[17] Some food allergies last a lifetime, while others appear and later disappear. The cause of food allergies is not known.

Today, an enormous number of people think they have food allergies. The February 1988 edition of *Consumer Reports* attributes the recent "boom" in food allergies to unorthodox allergy practitioners who diagnose (and treat) allergies where none are found by accepted techniques. In addition, people often mistake food intolerances for food allergies.

If you think that you have food allergies, see a board-certified allergist. She can give you skin tests to determine if you are truly allergic. If the test is negative, then it is highly unlikely that you are allergic. If it is positive, you may be allergic, but confirmation requires a history of allergic reactions or a controlled oral "challenge" with the suspect food under the supervision of a physician.

If you are allergic to a food (foods), your allergist will probably tell you to avoid it (them). Some people offer expensive shots for food allergies, but the American Academy of Allergy and Immunology maintains that these and related techniques have "no plausible rationale or immunologic basis."[18] Therefore, until more evidence supports these new treatments, you might do better to rely on the advice of a board-certified allergist and save your money.

Food *intolerances* do not provoke an immune response; however, the physical symptoms can be indistinguishable from allergy symptoms. For instance, the most common food intolerance is a lactose (milk sugar) intolerance, which is caused by a specific enzyme deficiency. Those who have a lactose intolerance typically suffer from diarrhea or stomach cramps after drinking milk or eating dairy products. Luckily, excellent alternatives are available, including lactaid milk, lactaid cottage cheese, soy milk, soy cheese, goat's milk, and goat's cheese. In addition, most people can avoid a negative reaction to milk products by taking the needed digestive enzyme, lactaid, in a tablet.

One can be, or become, intolerant to almost any food. Luckily, food intolerances often disappear or can be overcome over time. Frani Pollack, a nutritionist at the Geselle Institute, frequently works with people who suffer from food allergies and intolerances. She says that if a person stops eating the offending food for a period of time (a year is often sufficient), then the food can often be reintroduced in progressively larger amounts without provoking a response. Thus a great many food allergies and food intolerances are only *temporary*, especially if treated correctly.

Many food intolerances are mild enough that one need not give up the food completely. For instance, I have an intolerance to wine and champagne—they make me nauseous—but I find that if I limit myself to half a glass, I feel fine. I am also intolerant of caffeine, but, again, if I limit myself to one cup of coffee or tea, then I do not get sick. These kinds of mild intolerances need not stand in the way of spontaneous eating.

Many sufferers say that in times of stress and/or unhappiness, food intolerances become worse, while in "good times" the reactions lessen. Others have reported that when they are in good physical condition, their reactions are less severe or even absent. I do not know of any scientific evidence or explanation to back up these reports. Nonetheless, if you have mild or moderate food intolerances, you may want to do a self-test to discover if the same is true for you. Find a time when you can get plenty of sleep, eat very healthily, and exercise regularly. After three or four weeks of this "good living," try eating a little of an offending food and see how you feel. If your tolerance is higher, you will have found one more reason to live well on a regular basis!

If you have a severe reaction to a food(s), then it is a good idea to see an allergist or a nutritionist (who specializes in food intolerances) and avoid the food(s) completely. Pretend that it doesn't even exist (except to avoid it). Aside from unusual cases, people are allergic or highly intolerant to only a small number of foods, and these specific food limitations need not stand in the way of spontaneous eating. Simply focus on spontaneously eating the wide range of foods that *are* available to you.

If you have severe reactions to a wide variety of foods, or if you have a medical condition that strictly limits your food choices, I'm afraid that I have no easy solution. It will be much harder for you to develop spontaneous eating. The best you can do is to find as many *allowable* foods as you can and, again, focus on spontaneously eating those foods.

A close friend of mine has successfully learned to cope with a very wide variety of severe food intolerances without giving up on spontaneous eating. She recommends that you set aside two or three hours and go into a large supermarket with pen and paper. Go down every aisle reading labels, and make a list of everything you *can* eat. When you notice foods you have never had before, buy and try them. If you like a new food, add it to your list. Save this list. Stock your kitchen from it. And when you get to feeling that "there's nothing out there" for you, look at it again and see if you haven't temporarily forgotten about foods you like. Even if you

are allergic to (or intolerant of) many foods, you will probably find that there is still an amazing variety of delicious foods from which to choose.

ABOUT SUGAR

In my workshops I have repeatedly seen that some women can eat sugar (and sugary foods) without any significant problem, while others find that sugar leads to insatiable hunger and bingeing. Most people find that this problem disappears when an appropriate setpoint weight is maintained and dieters' mind-set has been overcome; however, I have known a few people who cannot seem to shake this reaction to sugar.

If you are struggling with a painful reaction to sugar, you have two reasonable alternatives. You can continue to eat sugar and simply work toward your goals with the hope that the problem will dissipate over time; or you can try to break free from sugar. If your reaction to sugar is only mild, then I recommend that you choose the former. However, if your reaction to sugar is severe, you may feel much better and progress in other areas more easily if you go "cold turkey."

If you are in the habit of eating large amounts of sugar on a daily basis, it will not be easy to break free from it. In fact, you will probably suffer from some withdrawal symptoms. Fatigue, depression, insatiability, and virtually uncontrollable urges for sweets are commonly experienced by people who have severe problems with sugar. Luckily, these withdrawal symptoms rarely last for more than four to seven days, after which you should feel much better. Once you get over this "hump," you will probably find that your cravings for sugar steadily decrease until you stop missing it.

I never needed to go through this painful process, because my reactions to sugar have never been severe. However, I have seen others do it and come out feeling that it was well worth the pain involved. Making this choice does not preclude spontaneous eating afterward. In fact, it can help because you will no longer have to struggle with disruptive and painful reactions to sugar as you relearn to eat in a natural way. Should you decide that you need to break free from sugar, I recommend that you do the following:

1. Get rid of all the sugar, nonnutritive sweeteners,* and sugary foods in your house or apartment.

2. Enlist two close friends or family members to "be there" for you when you find yourself going crazy for sugar. Whenever you get the craving, call or go see one of them instead of eating sugar.

3. For the first week, avoid social events that will bring you into contact with sugary foods. Plan your break from sugar at a time when this will not keep you from anything important.

4. Keep yourself as busy and involved as possible. Pack your days with interesting work and enjoyable play, leaving as little time for boredom as possible. Avoid watching unengrossing television, espe-

cially alone or with people who eat while they watch.

5. Try to find a food you can enjoy in place of sugar, particularly for the first week. Popcorn with a small glass of juice is a good option, since this snack will boost your blood sugar (but less drastically and more gradually than sugar) and satisfy hunger. Or, if you are not hungry enough for such a substantial snack, try a piece of fruit.

6. Be sure to eat sugar-free meals and snacks at regular intervals. Do not allow yourself to go hungry.

7. Try to get plenty of exercise. It will help keep your spirits up and may prevent sleeplessness.

8. If at first you don't succeed, try again. In fact, if you eat sugar after avoiding it for a number of days, try to get back to abstaining right away because all progress will not necessarily have been lost. You could be just a few days from the end of the intense withdrawal symptoms.

Luckily, most people do not have to go through anything this drastic. However, if you are one of the unlucky people who feel addicted and driven by large quantities of sugar, it may be worth trying to break free from it despite the cost in freedom and the pain of withdrawal. Furthermore, your complete abstinence from sugar may not have to be permanent. After you have made progress in other areas discussed in this book, you will probably be able to enjoy small amounts of sugar without any noticeable reaction.

* Nonnutritive sweeteners often cause cravings for sweets and should therefore be treated the same as sugar.

ABOUT EXERCISE

Workshop members invariably want to know how much I exercise. As with eating choices, *my* exercise habits are mostly irrelevant. Nonetheless, I will share my experiences with you.

When I was struggling to break free from my eating disorder, I used exercise as a way to fight off anxiety and destructive impulses. Since I was virtually overcome with both of these, I exercised for an hour almost every day. I knew it was obsessive, but it was the least destructive of my impulses, so it seemed reasonable to allow compulsive exercising for as long as I needed it.

After a few years, I was effortlessly maintaining a healthy weight and felt mostly free from diet/weight conflict. Therefore, I was able to exercise less without anxiety. Today I try to exercise three times a week, for between half an hour and an hour each time, depending on my schedule and my whim of the moment. I try to spread the exercise over the week, roughly every other day. This feels best because it gives my muscles recovery time between workouts.

My favorite forms of aerobic exercise at the moment include rapid walking in hilly areas with a friend, running (alone), stationary bicycle with a good novel, lap swimming, and aerobic dancing. (For other examples of aerobic exercise, see Chapter 3.)

I am extremely lucky in that I truly love my life. I love the balance I've found: the balance between relaxation and exercise, between work and play, between healthy eating and recreational eating, between loving companionship and being alone. Not long ago I did not have a happy or healthy balance in any of these areas. It is truly amazing how far we can all come toward living well, even after living very poorly and unhappily.

As you work through the following workbook pages, keep in mind that this is your real goal: to learn to live happily. Not to "control your eating" or to "get in shape"—these aren't the all-important goals in life. The important thing is that you find a way of life, a "life-style," that makes *you* feel good and happy. And your way is likely to be somewhat different, maybe very different, from my way. Try to feel utterly free to be who you are and to make the choices you want to make. It is your life.

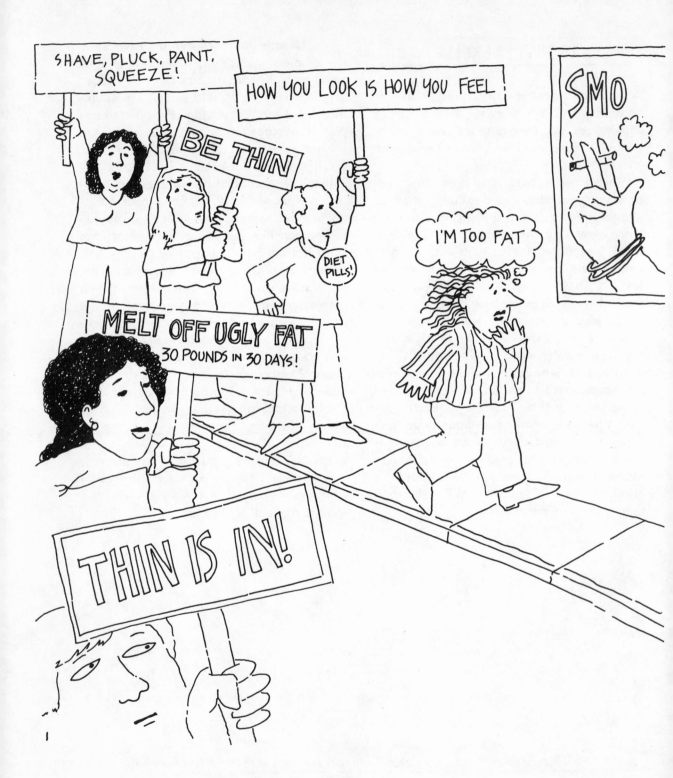

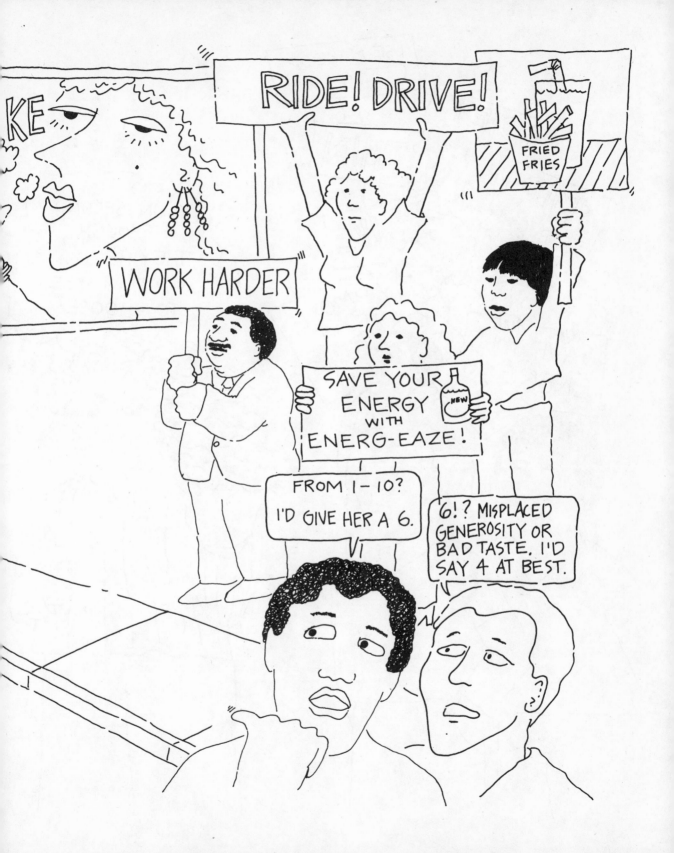

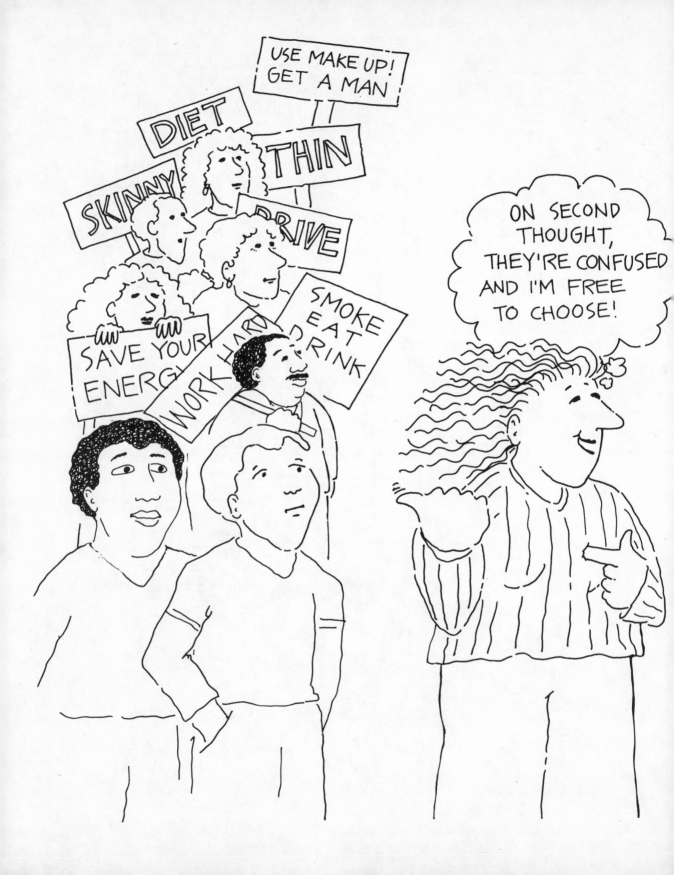

PERSONAL QUESTIONS:
EXPLORING AND ENVISIONING YOUR LIFE-STYLE

1. Describe your current eating habits and how you feel about them.

2. Do you want to develop a new vision of how you would like to eat? If so, why? How do you expect or hope that this will help you? (If not, skip ahead to the exercise questions.)

3. Make a list of the nutritious foods you would like to eat at home, using the food charts on pp. 178 through 180 as a guide. Put an H next to each of the habitual staple foods and a star next to all your favorite foods. (Do NOT include any food that seems to cause a negative reaction for you.)

NUTRITIOUS FOOD I LIKE TO EAT AT HOME

4. Are there any nutritional gaps in your list? In other words, if you ate solely from the preceding list of foods, could you eat in a well-balanced way? If not, how would you like to change this? Is it possible that you could add something that would fill in the gap(s)?

5. Make a list of nutritious foods you would like to eat away from home. Again, put an H next to each of the habitual staple foods and a star next to all your favorite foods.

NUTRITIOUS FOOD I LIKE TO EAT OUT

6. Are your lists of healthy food long and varied? Do you think that you could eat in a joyful, satisfying way if the *bulk* of your intake consisted of these foods? Why or why not?

7. Make a list of the not-so-nutritious or recreational foods you would like to eat at home. Put stars next to your favorites. Put an X next to any items that seem to cause negative reactions (allergic reactions or tiredness, headache, etc.).

Nutritional Guidelines and Spontaneity: Developing a Healthy Life-Style

```
┌─────────────────────────────────────────────────────┐
│          RECREATIONAL FOOD I LIKE TO EAT AT HOME      │
├─────────────────────────────────────────────────────┤
│                                                       │
│                                                       │
│                                                       │
│                                                       │
│                                                       │
│                                                       │
│                                                       │
└─────────────────────────────────────────────────────┘
```

8.   Make a list of the recreational foods you would like to eat away from home. Again, put stars next to your favorites and Xs next to foods that cause problems.

```
┌─────────────────────────────────────────────────────┐
│          RECREATIONAL FOOD I LIKE TO EAT OUT          │
├─────────────────────────────────────────────────────┤
│                                                       │
│                                                       │
│                                                       │
│                                                       │
│                                                       │
│                                                       │
│                                                       │
└─────────────────────────────────────────────────────┘
```

9. In your ideal vision, are there foods that you imagine yourself never (or virtually never) eating simply because the negative consequences (such as allergic reactions) aren't worth the eating pleasure? If so, what food(s)?

10. Are there foods you did not include on any of the preceding lists that you now eat? If so, why do you eat food you don't particularly like?

11. In your ideal vision, do you foresee any kind of line or difference between habitual eating (that is, foods you buy and eat on a regular basis) and other eating (foods you eat only occasionally)? Why or why not?

Nutritional Guidelines and Spontaneity: Developing a Healthy Life-Style

12.   Pretend that you are completely *free from your diet/weight conflicts*. Close your eyes and try to imagine buying food at the grocery store, cooking and eating at home, eating at other people's homes, eating out . . . in a way you consider life-supportive (that is, supportive of your health, well-being, and happiness). Now describe how you would stock your kitchen, how often and to what kinds of restaurants you would go, what you would eat (an overview), and how you would make your eating decisions.

13.   In this vision, do you picture yourself eating in a spontaneous and healthy way? Do you foresee comfortable eating patterns with some consistency but without rigidity? Why or why not?

14.   Do you picture yourself eating recreational food when you want to? Why or why not?

15.   Do you think your vision is realistic? Do you believe it is possible for you to enjoy your eating fully, feel satisfied by what you eat, and eat in a healthy way? Why or why not?

16.   In what ways do you benefit—not according to experts but according to your own experience—from exercise?

17.   Overall, do you consider regular exercise life-supportive for you? (If not, skip the rest of these questions.)

18.   Ideally, how much time would you like to spend exercising each week? Do you think you can meet that goal? Why or why not?

19. If your career (or some other personal circumstance) someday requires that you get very little exercise for a significant period of time, how well do you think you will be able to deal with it? How much does exercise affect your well-being, and how important is it in relation to other parts of your life?

20. What do you consider the "ideal" attitude toward exercise (for yourself)? In what ways will this attitude support your health and happiness? In what ways could this attitude hurt you, if at all?

21. During the next forty years, how much do you picture yourself exercising and why? When might you exercise more or less than at other times in your life and why?

9

REVIEWING OUR STEPS
TO FREEDOM

In Chapter 1 I asked that you reconceptualize your problem. You probably thought that you had a "weight problem," and I suggested that you had a painful preoccupation (and conflicts) with diet and weight. By now you have seen that this redefinition is more than a game with words. If you think your problem is solely a matter of body weight, then your goal is probably weight loss. However, if you know that your problem is a painful preoccupation with diet and weight (and associated destructive behavior), then your goal should be freedom from that preoccupation.

I am committed to treating our problem as a matter of conflict and preoccupation; however, I am well aware that the choice is difficult to make. We are all under tremendous pressure to believe that we have a "weight problem," and to treat it accordingly. The thin-is-in craze has given rise to an enormous number of books, companies, self-help groups, and other programs that claim to help people eat less, lose weight, and im-

prove their lives. Most of you have tried some of these programs. All of you will continue to hear about them in conversations and advertisements.

Working toward freedom from diet/weight conflict will be a constant challenge. Even after progressing a long way, you may (at times) feel discouraged and frightened by the choices you're making. If this happens and you find yourself drawn to the many "solutions" that offer so much, don't blame yourself. Even if you return to destructive ways of eating, you haven't "failed." Beware of applying reverse value judgments: "Oh I've been so *bad* lately—I'm dieting *again* even though I know it's destructive. What's wrong with me?"

What's "wrong" is that you're not a magician. You haven't been able to let go of your preoccupation as quickly as you would have liked. What's "wrong" is that the tremendous pressures to be thin at any cost are breaking you down. But *you are not bad.* You are perfectly fine. And you are doing the

Reviewing Our Steps to Freedom

best you can, which is always 100 percent good enough.

If you decide to use one of the many "solutions" on the market, choose carefully. Some can be used in conjunction with attempts to attain freedom from diet/weight conflict, while others cannot. Some will control your "symptoms" (such as bingeing, starving, and purging) better than others. Some have helpful elements even though they rest on faulty assumptions and potentially destructive goals. This is important to understand, both if you decide to use one (or more) of these programs, and if you want to understand and help others who use them.

FREQUENTLY OFFERED "SOLUTIONS" TO WEIGHT PROBLEMS

"Solution" #1: Weight-Loss Diets

Most people go on weight-loss diets because they think that their "weight problem" is caused by overeating. The solution seems obvious: eat less until a desired weight is attained and then avoid overeating in the future. The problem with this solution has been well documented by Bennett and Gurin in *The Dieter's Dilemma: Eating Less and Weighing More*, as well as in Chapter 3 of this book. Quite simply, our bodies have defense mechanisms that efficiently and consistently oppose our attempts to lose more than a certain amount of fat: they defend a setpoint weight that is, for the most part, an inherited physical trait.

Temporary weight-loss diets can be very satisfying. They allow us to take control of our diets and to enjoy *measurable* results, both of which tend to make us feel better about ourselves. Should you decide to go on a weight-loss diet sometime in the future, remember that you will be boosting your self-esteem in a temporary way. You may feel as though you're taking control of yourself and therefore feel more effective and strong. But unless this feeling allows you to take meaningful and useful action in other areas of your life, you will have attained very little. If you later experience the usual postdiet insatiability, bingeing, and rapid weight gain, try not to blame yourself. Try not to feel that you are "bad" while immersed in this part of the cycle. Even if you don't binge, you will probably regain the weight you lost (though at a slower rate). That is part of the "package deal" known as weight-loss dieting.

The negative effects of weight-loss diets have already been discussed at great length. The most important is: they usually produce destructive physical and psychological side effects. *Temporary weight-loss diets promote diet/weight preoccupation and eating disorders* without providing any lasting positive effects. They are probably the most harmful of all the pseudo-solutions we are so frequently encouraged to pursue.

"Solution" #2: Weight-Loss Pills

Given our medication-oriented society, it is not surprising that weight-loss pills are widely available. Every drugstore offers appetite suppressants (for relatively pain-free starvation) and diuretics (for artificially induced dehydration). A few charletan doctors prescribe potent stimulants ("uppers") so their patients lose weight *and* become addicted to physically and psychologically harmful drugs.

Appetite suppressants and other drugs can cause people to lose weight, but they do not promote permanent weight loss any more than weight-loss diets. Furthermore, these pills represent the ultimate expression of contempt for the human body. Those who market weight-loss drugs are saying, "Don't pay any attention to your body—silence it with pills." Their appeal is obvious: "It's quick, it's easy, and it's painless—just pop 'em in and watch what happens." What happens first is that people chemically alienate themselves from their bodies. Second, most people regain weight as soon as they stop taking pills because their body's defense mechanisms promptly return. In short, the only option more harmful than a weight-loss diet is probably a weight-loss diet with "diet pills." (Note: "diet pills" do not include antidepressant drugs, which may help bulimics.)

"Solution" #3: Programmed Eating

Eating according to an *explicit* diet (which specifies foods and amounts) is another "solution."[1] The content of the diet programs varies. However, they all have at least one thing in common: rigidity. No spontaneous eating is allowed. The goal is to follow an eating program without exception.

Programmed eating has helped many people break out of destructive eating patterns after other "solutions" failed. Unfortunately, it is not designed to *cure* eating disorders or diet/weight preoccupation. The underlying assumption is that "compulsive overeating" and associated problems are *incurable*—that the best you can hope to do is control symptoms. People who eat in this rigid way have given up on the possibility of spontaneous eating. They have also given up personal responsibility for what they eat.

It may seem contradictory to state that when people rigidly adhere to explicit diets they are, in effect, giving up responsibility and control; however, programmed eating simulates the release from eating decisions. When a person follows an explicit diet without question, the diet, rather than the individual, controls her eating.

Some programmed eaters are chronically underweight and underfed but don't know it. Their cycles of compulsive overeating and dieting developed through the pursuit of excessively low weights. Through programmed eating, they attain their self-destructive goal at a very high cost.

Despite all its flaws, programmed eating has provided many people with desperately needed relief, and this relief from torment should not be taken lightly. It is a fantastic accomplishment whenever someone who suffers from severe eating problems controls her symptoms. Ideally, adherence to the program becomes automatic, so that sufferers can focus on more important issues and tasks. "To eat or not to eat" stops being their focal issue. Consequently, many people are able to work on other problems (such as chronic loneliness and isolation) and thus build happier lives while eating in a programmed way.

Programmed eating can also be used, of course, as a temporary measure. Some sufferers may not want to give up spontaneous eating forever, but may need immediate relief from very destructive eating patterns. Programmed eating can be used as a resting place and stepping-stone toward freedom from diet/weight conflict. Once sufferers relearn how good it feels to eat in a more consistent—neither excessive nor insufficient—way, they may find it easier to normalize their eating.

It saddens me to see people use programmed eating as a permanent solution. Like Carolyn Jones, who watched her husband overcome compulsive bingeing and obesity through programmed eating (in *Diary of a Food Addict*), I mourn the personal loss of dietary freedom and all the social and personal pleasures that go along with it. Giving up dietary freedom means giving up not only certain pleasures, but spontaneity. We all need more pleasure and spontaneity in our lives—not less.

In short, this "solution" can be a constructive step for some people, but it is a sorry replacement for freedom. All those who control their symptoms through programmed eating deserve to go beyond: to free themselves of diet/weight conflict as well as from its symptoms.

"Solution" #4: Overeaters Anonymous

Overeaters Anonymous (OA) is a self-help organization based on the very well-known Alcoholics Anonymous (AA). Their twelve-step program to recovery from compulsive overeating mirrors AA's twelve-step program to recovery from alcoholism. Neither group seeks to "cure" their members' compulsive eating or alcoholism, but rather to help members "abstain from" or control their symptoms.

Overeaters Anonymous used to promote programmed eating; however, in 1987 they took steps to change that. Whereas they used to define abstention from compulsive overeating in terms of a rigid eating program, they now allow each member to define abstention for him/herself. Whereas they used to distribute a food plan called the "gray sheet" and recommend weighing and measuring all food to be eaten, they now offer no food plans or other specific guidelines for eating. Instead, OA recommends that members seek recovery as they see fit, using the twelve steps.

The steps are very spiritual in nature. In summary, they require that one (a) recognize and openly admit to being "powerless over food,"[2] (b) turn oneself over to a Higher Power (God), and (c) take a moral inventory of oneself on an ongoing basis, again seeking God's help for positive change. Thus OA members seek recovery from compulsive overeating through a spiritual awakening.

Without a doubt, OA has helped an enormous number of people, not only with compulsive overeating but with anorexia and bulimia as well. It is an excellent organization, and the twelve steps can be very effective. Their decision to move away from rigid food plans was a good one, as it will allow OA members to move further toward true recovery, rather than just the control of symptoms.

My only qualm about OA is that they continue to promote the idea that the sufferer is powerless and that compulsive overeating and related disorders are incurable—

that one's Higher Power can control the symptoms, but one can never be completely free of the "illness." This is simply untrue. Anorexics, bulimics, and compulsive overeaters are not powerless, and they *can* break completely free. They don't have to settle for the control of symptoms. Show me a sufferer who truly believes that a complete recovery or "cure" is impossible, and I'll show you a sufferer who will never recover—until she changes her mind and comes to believe that she *can!*

"Solution" #5: Permanent Change of Diet

Three dietary changes are enough to decrease most people's setpoints: the elimination of simple sugars (such as white and brown sugar, honey, syrups, etc.) and the drastic reduction of fats and *processed* grains (such as white flour). If these three changes are maintained, most people can eat as much as they want, promote good health, and permanently reduce their setpoints.[3]

This is not to say that everyone can become healthy *and skinny* through this kind of diet. Some people's "low setpoints" are higher than most people's "high setpoints." A naturally fat person would lose weight by making the above changes, but her body type wouldn't change. She would just become thinner than before.

Most people find it very difficult to maintain *drastic* changes in diet because strong influences oppose that choice. Most prepared foods (in supermarkets and restaurants) include sugar and/or a lot of fat and/or processed grain. Most recipes include

those ingredients. The foods offered at parties tend to include those ingredients. Many of the foods we have been brought up on, and love, include those ingredients. . . . In short, we would have to shop differently, cook differently, and avoid a large proportion of the foods we are offered by other people. Anyone who eats institutional food, or is very socially active, or lives and eats with people who want to eat in a more relaxed way, will find these dietary changes difficult to maintain.

Nonetheless, I believe that *gradual* dietary changes can help many of those who suffer from diet/weight conflict. It is essential to avoid embarking on a strict "program" of eating that will feel like just another form of dreaded deprivation, but this is often possible. The key is to be patient and avoid focusing on weight loss as the goal or reason behind your dietary changes. Instead, make the changes, slowly but surely, for your well-being, health, and happiness. Be sure to enjoy eating, avoid being fanatical or rigid about the choices you make, eat in harmony with your hunger and satiation, and try to keep dieters' mind-set from creeping into your efforts. In this way, permanent dietary changes can be a helpful part of a chronic dieter's, anorexic's, or bulimic's efforts to break free.

"Solution" #6: Exercise Programs

Exercise programs are among the best of the pseudosolutions. They can promote health, well-being, and a more instrumental (rather than purely ornamental) body view. Unfortunately, many exercise programs cater to people's desire to "improve" their appearance through weight loss. Participants are encouraged to focus on how many inches and pounds they can lose (or redistribute). These programs are often more harmful than helpful because they increase people's obsessions with appearance and weight.

Luckily, exercise programs need not focus on appearance at all and can therefore be 100 percent beneficial. Through exercise, people can find new ways of enjoying themselves while simultaneously improving their health, and thereby gain a new kind of appreciation for their bodies.

Conclusions About the "Solutions"

Whenever people try a new weight-loss program, they tend to respond as promised—at first. No matter how faulty the underlying theory or how ultimately damaging the program, early results are often gratifying to the desperate dieter. Envision the "ultimate" program: clients receive "new," "extensively tested and proven" weight-loss schemes on a regular basis. Just as one scheme is about to stop working, the client is given a new one! The content of the programs themselves is not particularly important. Their purpose is to excite and motivate the clients—to give them some hopeful plan to work with and believe in. New diet books and weight-loss clinics are constantly coming out and "succeeding" on this principle.

Nearly all of this "success" has been *temporary*, for these "solutions," at most, control or mask the *symptoms* of the problem. None cures the problem itself. The vast majority of people who lose weight rapidly gain it back. At best, they end up where they started. At worst, they emerge with lower self-esteem and a more intense diet/weight obsession.

My preoccupation with diet and weight increased with every cycle of weight loss and gain. At first, dieting was like a game—I almost enjoyed starving myself and losing weight. However, the game soon lost its charm. Every time I tried a new "solution," I lost weight, gained it back, and emerged more preoccupied with diet and weight than ever before. The more preoccupied I became, the harder I worked to solve my "weight problem." By the time I thought I had solved it, weight control had become the core of my life and self-esteem.

Does this sound familiar? Are you tormenting yourself now? I have written this book to say that we have another choice. We don't have to obsess about our bodies. We don't have to struggle and torture ourselves in the pursuit of slenderness. Instead, we can attain freedom from diet/weight conflict and fight the epidemic of eating disorders.

Most self-help books say: "Here's The Solution to your problem! It's quick, it's easy, and you're going to love it!" The truth is that the resolution of diet/weight conflict and preoccupation is rarely quick or easy. Many complex forces cause our preoccupation, and many of them are relentless external pressures that are impossible to avoid. Consequently, those of us who want to be free of the diet/weight obsession are faced with a lot of work. *We must undermine the causes of our preoccupation* by eliminating those we can eliminate, and learning to live with those we cannot.

CHOOSING SOMETHING NEW: A SUMMARY OF PERSONAL WORK

It is tempting to believe that if we understand why we suffer from a diet/weight obsession, our understanding alone will set us free. Unfortunately, it rarely works that way. Studying eating disorders, nutrition, and other related subjects can even intensify our problem. We need to understand why we are preoccupied with diet and weight in order to know what to do about it. But then we have to *stop studying it and start undermining the causes that drive us.*

The road to freedom from diet/weight conflict *begins* with understanding, but the rest requires deliberate action. We must change our attitudes, feelings, behavior, and environment. We must begin a gradual process of working through, reaching out, growing, and letting go. As you read the following review of suggested personal work, notice the items that speak to you most. You don't have to eliminate every cause of diet/weight conflict in order to free yourself from it. Focus your efforts in accordance with your own needs and judgment.

Expanding Body Appreciation

In order to go beyond our culture's narrow definition of beauty, we need to develop an appreciation for the beauty of all body types. We have learned to see the beauty of slenderness because it is constantly idealized. We can learn to see the beauty of fatness by studying and looking for it:

1. Learn from the artists who have idealized relatively fat women by going to see their work in museums, collecting and displaying prints of their work in your home, and reading enlightened commentaries. Some famous artists to look for include Titian (Tiziano Vecellio), Rubens, Renoir, Giorgione, Manet, and Tintoretto. Also look for contemporary feminist art that celebrates big women.

2. Look at the big people around you, noting the full and graceful curves of their beautiful bodies. (If someone catches you staring at him/her, be sure to smile and say hello.)

3. If you know (or meet) someone who is attracted to fat women, ask that person to tell you about who she finds beautiful (in the streets, in pictures, or among the people you know) and why. You can learn a lot by finding out what she finds so beautiful.

4. Learn to appreciate the wonderful "feel" of fat people. Soft fullness is delightful for hugging and touching!

5. Choose to get to know and love some fat people. Spending time with fat people who are at peace with their bodies is especially gratifying and helpful.

6. Take advantage of any opportunity to visit countries where fatness is still idealized, such as India or Nepal.

In addition to undermining the idealization of slenderness, remember that weight loss and slenderness are not all they're cracked up to be. When you are exposed to propaganda that presents weight loss as the solution to all your problems, remind yourself that it's not true. Slenderness does not guarantee happiness, and fatness does not guarantee unhappiness—far from it. Also recall what you know about setpoint theory. Take a critical look at the advertisement (or whatever) in light of what you have learned.

Loving People of All Sizes

Contradict all three forms of fattism in your daily life: fattist feelings and thoughts within yourself, other people's expressions of fattism, and fattism in the media. To let go of your own fattism:

1. Train yourself to appreciate and respect people of every size and shape.

2. Beware of stereotyping fat people. Remember that fat people are *not* any less intelligent, less capable, less well-adjusted, or more gluttonous than thin people.

3. Make sure you are not avoiding fat people in any way.

4. Don't tell jokes that abuse fat people.

5. Don't assume that fat people would be healthier or "better off" if they lost weight.

6. Don't assume that fat people want to lose weight.

7. Join an organization that promotes "fat liberation" (see Resources, p. 229).

8. In short, accord fat people the same appreciation and respect that you accord thinner people. Be on the lookout: it takes years to eliminate your own fattism completely.

Others' fattism represents a constant challenge because fat people have become one of the favored scapegoats in our society. Most people feel justified in their fattism and don't recognize it as a destructive prejudice. Try to point out and object to others' fattist comments and behavior in an understanding and unaggressive way. If people insist upon maintaining their fattism, feel free to avoid their company.

Fattism in the media, on the other hand, is impossible to avoid. You must learn to recognize and reject each fattist message in order to avoid being brainwashed. Think of ways to protest. For instance, write to offending advertisers and networks. Your complaints may have more power than you expect because "sellers" cannot afford to alienate buyers. The National Association to Aid Fat Americans (NAAFA) organizes campaigns against offensive advertising and discrimination. See Resources for more information, and get involved!

Undermining Objectification

Both expanding your appreciation of the human body (to include fat people) *and* opposing human objectification may seem contradictory. After all, one part of learning to see the beauty of fatness is looking at many fat people as aesthetic objects. However, we can appreciate and enjoy people's physical beauty and still *treat* people as complete human beings. We can value their behavior and feelings more than their appearance. Undermine objectification:

1. Do not objectify yourself by continually scrutinizing yourself in mirrors, windows, etc.

2. When people objectify others (by rating their appearance, for example), explain

why it bothers you and ask that they stop.

3. Avoid those who insist upon objectifying people.

4. When you watch television or go to see a movie, look out for shows, commercials, and films that present people as aesthetic objects. Notice the mechanics of the objectification and how it affects you.

5. Avoid beauty contests and body-building competitions.

6. Avoid other obvious sources of objectification such as pornography and sexist films.

Developing an Instrumental Body View

We have learned to see our bodies as ornaments because we are barraged with objectification. As you undermine objectification, you can replace your ornamental body view with a more instrumental body view:

1. Do not wear uncomfortable clothing and shoes for the sake of appearance. (Be especially careful to avoid clothing that is too tight.)

2. Focus on how you feel (more than on how you look).

3. When you exercise, focus on enjoyment, coordination, and endurance rather than on calories burned or resulting changes in appearance.

4. In general, choose physical pleasure and avoid physical discomfort whenever possible. For instance, if you suffer from

menstrual cramps, find a treatment that will lessen or eliminate the discomfort. Also spend time enjoying your sexuality (alone or otherwise).

5. Practice appreciating your body for the ways in which it serves you well. Are you healthy? Are you energetic? Can you move around easily? How does your body help you enjoy life?

Relearning Spontaneous Eating

If you have been struggling to control your diet and weight for a long time, then you probably think like a chronic dieter, which virtually guarantees that you will suffer from diet/weight preoccupation. In order to stop thinking like a dieter, you must stop treating yourself like one. You must stop weight-loss dieting and relearn to eat spontaneously:

1. Never deprive yourself of something you really want to eat: eat and enjoy it fully. Be pleased with yourself for knowing what you wanted and fulfilling your desire.

2. Never force yourself to eat something you don't want. If someone's feelings seem to be at stake, just be as kind and reassuring as you can be.

3. Make physical comfort a constant goal. Always try to eat exactly the amount of food that will please you most and make you feel best. Avoid feeling "starved" or "stuffed."

4. Be aware that you *choose* what you eat. You are in control of your own choices. If you find yourself thinking, "I shouldn't be eating this," stop eating

for a moment. Remind yourself that if you really want that food, then you deserve to have and enjoy it. Ask yourself if you *want* to eat the food in front of you. If the answer is "yes," reassure yourself: "I really want this, so I'm going to eat and enjoy it." Enjoy.

5. Recall how you felt *before* you became concerned about diet and weight. Try to recreate that feeling.

6. Do not count calories.

7. Try not to think in terms of "good" and "bad" food or "good" and "bad" eating.

8. Remember that how and what you choose to eat has nothing to do with your value. You are a good person. Nothing you can choose to eat (or avoid) has the power to make you "bad," and nothing you can choose to eat (or avoid) has the power to make you "better."

9. Do not weigh yourself. You are probably in the habit of using your weight as a measurement of your value and as a source of motivation for self-starvation. Don't play with that chain reaction!

10. As you learn to eat spontaneously, don't blame yourself for your difficulties and setbacks. You are in a process of dramatic change. Appreciate your victories and learn from your setbacks. Remember that you are always doing the best you can, which is 100 percent good enough.

Developing Life-Supportive Values

Without knowing it, we all try to fulfill the destructive and inconsistent demands of our social system. Those efforts leave us feeling ineffective and bad about ourselves. You can undermine hurtful, dehumanizing values by developing and clarifying your own values:

1. Examine the human characteristics you value. Try to prevent definitions of "femininity" and "masculinity" from prescribing the characteristics you value for yourself and for other people.

2. Examine your goals. Try to prevent sex roles from prescribing your goals and way of life. Remember that you are free to choose who you are and what you do.

3. Examine your choices, past and present. Notice the ways in which others' expectations and values have directed your life. Take action, as needed, to make your choices fully *your own*.

4. Consider whether you suffer from a "Cinderella complex." Remember that *you* must instill your life with purpose, meaning, and satisfaction. A lover or spouse can't do it for you.

5. Examine your values and goals regarding relationships.

Learning to Love Ourselves

Almost everyone needs to develop a stronger and more positive sense of self. Up until now you have probably tried to earn self-respect and the respect of others through achievement. If you are a hard-core achiever, you know that this method doesn't work.

Achievement alone does not provide positive self-esteem. Try some other methods:

1. Learn to respect and accept yourself unconditionally. Remember that you deserve to feel good about yourself, and your life will improve when you treat yourself well.

2. Infuse your life with love for other people. Learn to be as loving as you can be, both by studying and practicing that art. Do not isolate yourself! Remember that isolation only breeds dissatisfaction with yourself and your life. Initiate contact despite your fears.

3. Replace negative "self-talk" (judgmental reprimands and criticism) with positive "self-talk" (nonjudgmental understanding and appreciation). Appreciate yourself without reservation.

4. Let go of perfectionism. Remember that perfection is a self-defeating impossibility. Instead of striving for perfection, know that you are always doing the best you can. Remember that you deserve to be proud of yourself and your efforts no matter what.

5. Let go of constant comparison and competition. Remember that you do not need to be or "do" better than anyone else in order to be a worthwhile person.

6. Look into your past for sources of low self-esteem. Think about messages you were given as a child about your worth (or relative worth). Once you understand how you were taught to have low self-esteem, you may find it easier to change. At the same time, remember that insight doesn't automatically pro-

duce positive self-esteem. You must change what you think and do.

7. Look for new ways to experience and practice self-reliance. This *doesn't* mean that you should isolate yourself. Just try something new by yourself—something that both excites and scares you.

8. Remember that you must have life-supportive values and goals in order to feel good about yourself. As previously discussed, this will require work.

Gaining Cooperation from Family and Friends

Your family and friends live in the same culture that has led you so far astray from a positive relationship with food, your body, and yourself. Consequently, you can expect to encounter virtually every destructive influence within your most important relationships. Loved ones may pressure you to be thin, to follow misguided programs, to accept their values as your own, etc. Loved ones may also objectify you and others and promote fattism. It can be tempting to let comments and suggestions slide by even when you know they hurt you. Be careful. Don't allow loved ones to hold you back if you can teach them to be supportive.

Work to communicate with your friends and family members with as much openness, love, and understanding as you can muster. Give them a chance to talk about their own pain around diet and weight. If they love you, then they will want to be good to you. Your job is to make sure that they know the difference between helpful and hurtful behavior. Ask them to read this

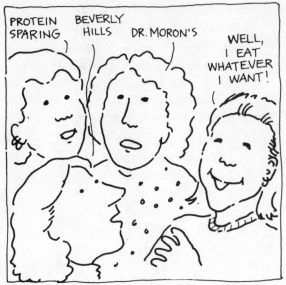 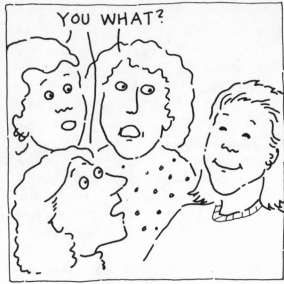

book. Explain the ways in which they are hurting you, but also say that you know they don't mean any harm. Ask for the kind of support you need—don't expect them to know your needs without being told.

When people don't respond well, try to be patient. Persist to whatever extent you think best and remember that people need time to learn new attitudes and behavior. If someone is particularly resistant to change and it is possible to avoid that person altogether, feel free to make that choice. Your relationships are very important, but your health and happiness are more important. If a certain relationship is very destructive and you feel unable to change it, you may need to leave it (temporarily or permanently, depending on the person and situation).

Choosing Your Life-Style

In order to be completely free of diet/weight conflict, you must maintain a comfortable (setpoint) weight, more or less effortlessly, and feel good about it. You cannot carry on a continual battle with your body and be at peace with your body at the same time. You know that from experience.

You have inherited a certain body type, and you probably have a pretty good idea of what type you have. You may not be able to estimate your setpoint weight range very accurately, but you probably know whether you are naturally very thin, very fat, or somewhere in between. In order to be free of diet/weight conflict, you need to accept your body type and fulfill your body's needs.

Here's where things get a little more complicated. Setpoint weight is affected by life-style—by the kinds of food you eat and the amount of exercise you get. If you eat fatty and sugary foods on a regular basis and choose a sedentary life-style (as most Americans do), then your setpoint will be higher (and you may be less comfortable and less healthy) than if you ate less fat and sugar and exercised more. If that is the life-style that pleases you most, fine. Enjoy! If not, then you can develop a different life-style. In any case, choose the one that will make *you* feel best. Don't necessarily choose the one mom and dad demonstrated, or the one your friends have chosen, or the one that will make you thinnest or fattest . . . but the one you really want.

One spring I came home from college and discovered that my parents had begun to eat in a completely different way. Neither had ever been on a weight-loss diet nor worried about weight, but my father had developed a minor health problem that could be reversed through substantial dietary restrictions. My parents changed their eating habits almost overnight and have maintained the changes ever since. That spring my mother said, "I can't understand why people find it hard to diet—it's so *easy* to change the way you eat!"

Why was it so easy for my parents to make enormous dietary changes? First of all, neither of them was trying to lose weight. Second, the changes were motivated by health, which they value highly. Third, they usually ate at home (both before and after the changes). And finally, they never attempted to deny their hunger. They were supposed to eat as much as they wanted; hence, they never went hungry.

In general, people find it hard to "diet" because they try to eat too little and pursue a weight that is below their setpoints. Their bodies respond with relentless defenses, one of which is intense hunger. From now on, avoid the pursuit of a certain weight like the plague. Seek a life-style that includes a way of eating and amounts of exercise that you enjoy; then accept the setpoint weight it promotes. Beware of the common and dangerous mistake of choosing a goal weight and then trying to attain that weight through changes in life-style. There is a profound difference between (a) choosing a weight and then seeking a life-style that will maintain it, and (b) choosing a supportive life-style and accepting the resulting weight. The former is likely to promote diet/weight obsession and dissatisfaction; the latter is likely to promote personal freedom and satisfaction.

Onward and Upward

We can all revolutionize our behavior and attitudes toward our bodies, our hunger, our eating, and ourselves. We can learn that thin people aren't better than fat people and learn to appreciate and celebrate the endless variety of human shapes and sizes. *Then* we can understand our epidemic of "weight problems" very differently: as an epidemic of diet/weight conflict, preoccupation, and associated self-abuse. The question will no longer be "How can we all make ourselves look the same (read: slender)?" The question will be "How can we all learn to love our bodies and ourselves, and treat our bodies and ourselves well?"

The time has come to stop focusing on diet and weight. Instead, we need to replace our preoccupation with ideas and tasks that will support our personal development. We must replace perfectionism and self-hatred with unconditional self-acceptance and appreciation. We must replace purely ornamental body views with more instrumental body

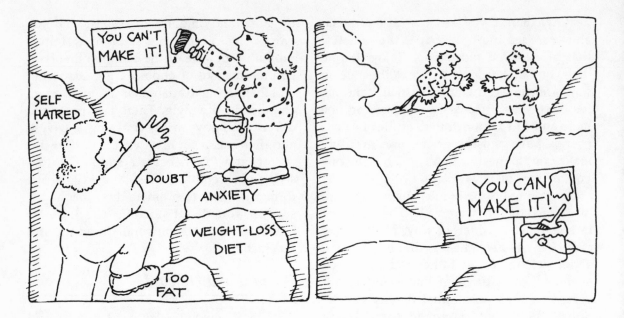

views. We must replace chronic dieting with spontaneous eating. We must stop using bathroom scales as indices to health, personal value, and progress. None of these changes can happen overnight, but they can happen. You can make them happen.

Toward this end, I have shared knowledge, personal work, and goals that have helped me let go of my own preoccupation with diet and weight. I have also encouraged you to develop your own answers. You need a new vision of your eating, yourself, and your life. Clearly, if I (or someone else) provided this vision, it couldn't act as *your* new vision of you, because it would be someone else's vision of you.

This book is full of ideas and information. However, I have helped people simply by explaining why *weight-loss dieting is harmful rather than beneficial*. If you put down this book having learned that basic fact and no other, you may have learned enough to let go of your preoccupation. A dear friend, Kate, has come a long way on that basis. She was a full-figured, large-hipped woman who had been a chronic dieter for as long as she could remember. One day I explained why weight-loss dieting was harmful rather than helpful and suggested that she try to eat spontaneously instead. She promptly rejected this idea, declaring that if she stopped dieting, she would surely become enormous. I let it drop.

A few years later, Kate told me that she never dieted anymore. Her weight was stabler and lower as a result, and she no longer felt deprived and hungry. She said that our conversation about dieting had been responsible for this turnaround. She had let my ideas shift around in her mind for a while and then acted upon them despite her fears.

Needless to say, my criticism of weight-loss dieting didn't provide a miraculous cure

—Kate cured herself. She developed her own visions and fulfilled them in her own way. This is as it must be for every person who suffers from diet/weight preoccupation. All you need is a little knowledge to counteract the propaganda and myths, loving support from people, and your own creative vision and energy. You are beautiful and capable and loving. You have the power to make your own choices—choices that will support your happiness and health.

A few months ago I went to a concert where a talented musician sang a celebration of "coming into her size" as a "big-boned woman."[4] The entire audience responded with approving cheers and applause. Last year I saw a fashion show of big women modeling beautiful clothes. Just the other day a former chronic dieter told me that her previous obsession with diet and weight seems alien to her now.

We are gradually changing ourselves and our society, and I'm glad to be a part of it. If you long for freedom from diet/weight conflict, then you, too, have become a part of it. Your longing for freedom may not be as strong as your longing to be model thin—not yet, anyway—but it's there and it's growing. It is a wonderful seed that has been planted, much as that first destructive seed—the thought "I am too fat"—was planted some time ago. This new seed can grow roots and branches to overwhelm the old one.

We're getting tired of draining ourselves and our lives in the pursuit of destructive goals. We're beginning to notice how everyone, ourselves included, encourages self-starvation, fattism, and thus diet/weight conflict and eating disorders. But more important, we're starting to see glimpses of something better: appreciation of the human body in every size and shape, the joy of spontaneous eating, self-acceptance, physical comfort, good health, and a life of loving.

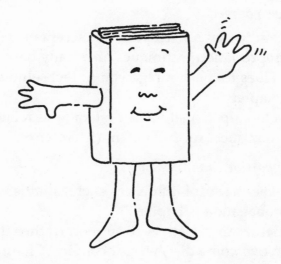

Reviewing Our Steps to Freedom

STEPS TO FREEDOM

Step 1: Learn to Be Good to Your Body

Understand your body's needs and defenses (Chapter 2), and learn to respect your physical integrity (Chapters 2–4, 8).

Step 2: Revise What "Thin" and "Fat" Mean to You

    a. Reject fattism: appreciate and respect people of every size and shape (Chapters 3, 10), including yourself (Chapter 5).
    b. Stop idealizing slenderness and slender people (Chapter 3).
    c. Expand your appreciation of the human body: learn to see beauty in all sizes (Chapters 3, 10).

Step 3: See People as Human Beings (Not Objects)

Learn to see and treat all people (including yourself) as *human beings* who have opinions, values, goals, feelings, intelligence, talents, etc., rather than as mere aesthetic objects (Chapter 3).

Step 4: Overcome and Replace Dieters' Mind-Set

Relearn to *listen* to your body and to eat spontaneously (Chapter 4).

Step 5: Learn to Love Yourself

    a. Strive for unconditional self-respect and acceptance (Chapter 5).
    b. Practice self-appreciation techniques on a daily basis (Chapter 5).
    c. Reject sexist values that encourage you to feel selfless, helpless, and inadequate (Chapter 6).
    d. Examine/develop a personal value system (and related goals) that will support your quest for fulfillment (Chapter 6).

Step 6: Create a Supportive Environment

    a. Openly contradict harmful influences such as fattism, sexism, and weight-loss propaganda (Chapter 7).
    b. Teach your friends and relatives to support (rather than undermine) your efforts to overcome diet/weight conflict (Chapters 7, 10).

Step 7: Develop a Supportive Life-style

Learn how your environment is affecting your life-style. Sort through your options and experiment. Gradually develop a way of eating and a pattern of exercise that support your quest for happiness and good health (Chapter 8).

FINAL QUESTIONS:
YOUR GOALS AND PLANS

1. Specify and discuss at least three of the most helpful concepts you have learned from this book. How have these concepts helped you? How might they help you in the future?

2. Make a list of goals you would like to pursue right away in order to work toward freedom from diet/weight conflict and greater life satisfaction.

3. What resources do you have to help you with the work toward these goals? What do you want to do first?

10

FOR SUFFERERS' LOVED ONES: OFFERING SUPPORT

In order to help someone who suffers from a diet/weight obsession (and/or an eating disorder), you must learn about its causes and stop participating in those causes. Reading this book is one good way to begin. This chapter provides an overview of ways in which you can become an ally to someone who is suffering from conflicts with diet and weight.

Before you try to use the rest of this chapter, it is essential that you read at least Chapters 1–4, 8, and 9 (you can skip the workbook pages). Without having read these chapters, you will not understand the reasons behind the suggestions that follow. If you don't understand the "why," you won't want to struggle with the "how." Your insufficient understanding of the problem would thus keep you from working toward helpful change. Go back and read these chapters now if you haven't done so already.

If your loved one is underweight, purging

(via self-induced vomiting, laxatives, or diuretics), or very depressed or upset, *encourage her to get professional help.* Most sufferers cannot overcome such severe problems by themselves (even with your help). They need individual and/or group therapy. If your eating-disordered loved one is your son, daughter, or spouse, then it is likely that family therapy will be needed, particularly if she/he still lives with you. You may also want to read *Surviving an Eating Disorder: New Perspectives and Strategies for Family and Friends* (see Resources, p. 241).

As a rule, try to take an unobtrusively supportive and loving role in your loved one's efforts to overcome her problem. *You cannot cure your loved one—she has to do it herself.* You can gently encourage constructive attitudes and behavior and be open to requests for support. However, the most helpful thing you can do is "clean up your own act." Most people who have been brought up in the Western world encourage diet/weight obsessions without knowing it. You probably do, too.

We know that the following influences promote diet/weight obsessions and eating disorders: objectification (the treatment of people as aesthetic objects), slender aesthetic ideals, the idealization of slender people, fattism (prejudice against fatness and fat people), the promotion of weight-loss programs, and popular myths about diet and weight control. Virtually everyone takes part in these harmful influences and thereby encourages diet/weight obsession and eating disorders. In order to encourage health and well-being instead, we must replace our harmful behavior.

It's difficult to change attitudes and habits. Such change demands motivation, clear goals, an effective strategy, and hard work. Before you determine your goals and strategy, assess your motivation. Ask yourself, "Am I truly motivated to promote health and well-being rather than diet/weight obsession and eating disorders?"

ASSESSING YOUR MOTIVATION

1. Why do you want to promote health and well-being rather than diet/weight preoccupation and eating disorders? Whom are you hoping to help? Why do you want to help?

2. How much do you care about the person (or people) you mentioned above? Do you care enough to make personal sacrifices (of at least time and energy)?

3. How much time are you willing to devote to personal goals (in order to help)? For example, is it worth ten minutes of your time each day? More? Less?

4. Are you willing to examine your beliefs, attitudes, and behavior with an open mind, or are you determined to hold fast to your past assumptions in order to appear "right?"

SPECIFIC RECOMMENDATIONS: A SUMMARY

In order to promote health and well-being rather than diet/weight conflict and eating disorders, strive to follow the dos and don'ts listed below.

Dos

1. *Do* your best to understand the causes of diet/weight obsession.

2. *Do* examine your aesthetic ideals. Do you idealize slenderness? Do you encourage your loved one to feel that she should be thin? If so, try to eliminate these harmful messages and expectations.

3. *Do* encourage healthy and spontaneous eating. Be a good example: eat in a relaxed and enjoyable way and do not voice worries or concerns regarding how much you eat or weigh.

4. *Do* appreciate your loved one fully for all she is and does. Every quality and action that is of greater value than appearance should be spoken of more than appearance.

5. *Do* let your loved one direct her own life. Respect her choices. Express your interest, support, opinions, and feelings, but don't be controlling or judgmental.

6. *Do* encourage an active life-style *for fun, health, and well-being.* Share activities such as walking, cycling, and dancing. However, *do not try to enforce an active life-style or make your loved one feel bad about inactivity.* Remember that *whether or not she exercises is not a moral issue.* She is *not* "good" when she exercises regularly and "bad" when she doesn't. Make your behavior reflect this understanding.

7. *Do* encourage your loved one to appreciate her body as a capable and integral part of herself (rather than as an aesthetic object).

8. *Do* encourage personal development by sharing thoughts and feelings about values, philosophy, and goals.

9. *Do* comment on aspects of health, personality, and appearance that are *positively* affected by spontaneous eating and/or weight gain. (If you let your loved one guess, she may assume the worst.)

10. *Do* help your loved one create a supportive environment:

    (a) Avoid movies and other media that contain especially heavy doses of objectification.

    (b) Spend time with people who do *not* encourage diet/weight conflict through objectification, fattism, sexism, etc.

    (c) Teach relatives and friends to avoid conversations and behavior that support diet/weight conflict.

(d) Criticize anything you see and hear that encourages diet/weight conflict.

11. *Do* examine your attitudes about eating. Do you ever talk about food or eating habits in terms of "good" and "bad"? Remember that food is not a *moral* issue. Avoid moralizing about food and encourage others to do the same.

12. *Do* examine your attitudes toward fatness and fat people. Try to eliminate your own fattism and reject (question and oppose) the fattism you observe.

13. *Do* learn as much as you can about the physiology of weight loss and gain. Challenge current myths about diet and weight.

14. *Do* encourage your loved one to love and appreciate herself unconditionally. Discourage self-criticism and competitiveness. Your loved one does not need to be "better than" others in order to be a special and worthwhile person. Make sure that what you say and do conveys that assumption.

15. *Do* encourage and support your loved one's efforts to overcome his/her diet/weight obsession. No one cures herself overnight. Make sure your loved one knows that you have faith in her even when she may seem to be failing.

Don'ts

1. *Don't* try to control, manipulate, or monitor your loved one's diet. Your diet is your concern, and your loved one's diet is her concern. That doesn't mean you shouldn't care about whether or not your loved one is eating in a self-destructive way. It means that you *must not try to control, or be judgmental about, your loved one's eating choices.*

2. *Don't* try to control or manipulate your loved one's actions, goals, or opinions (except through supportive discussion and debate when appropriate).

3. *Don't* praise, criticize, or comment on other people's appearance unless you have a constructive reason for doing so. When you focus on people's appearance, you encourage your loved one to focus (and worry about) her appearance—something she already does too much.

4. *Don't* criticize your loved one except in small, constructive doses, combined with loving appreciation.

5. *Don't* express or encourage slender aesthetic ideals.

6. *Don't* make fattist comments.

7. *Don't* express or encourage an ornamental body view.

8. *Don't* use the terms "good food" or "bad food," and don't ever say, "I (or she) was good (or bad) today," in order to characterize eating behavior.

9. *Don't* admire weight-loss dieting or rigidly controlled eating.

10. *Don't* admire obsessive exercising.

11. *Don't* talk like a dieter. For example, don't talk about weight, diet, or calories as dieters so often do.

12. *Don't* encourage perfectionism.

Your loved one needs loving support and freedom to deal with her problem and life as she sees fit. This is no different from what all people need: loving support and freedom to think and do as they choose. However, you will need to think carefully about what you say and do in order to help your loved one end her preoccupation with diet and weight. You need not take it to an extreme—don't act as though you're walking on eggshells—but do your best to cultivate attitudes, expectations, and behavior that will support your loved one's efforts to free herself from the diet/weight obsession.

When a loved one develops a serious problem, relatives and friends sometimes feel resentful and put out. "Why did this have to happen? Everything was just fine before this happened!" This reaction is understandable but unhelpful. Try to conceive of the difficulty in a positive way. Be glad that you are finding ways to improve important relationships. Realize that you and your loved one can *both* benefit from more communication. Realize that you and she can benefit from trying to understand and support each other more than you have in the past. What an exciting opportunity! Most people would do well to try to improve the important relationships in their lives. Unfortunately, many fail to do so because they do not see the need or do not know how to undertake the process.

Attitudes and behavior that support diet/weight conflict come very naturally to most of us. It takes time and effort to eliminate long-held destructive attitudes and behavior. Beware of underestimating your influence. When in doubt, ask your loved one how you can be most helpful. Discuss your feelings and needs as well as hers. Denial of problems and anxieties is not likely to help anyone. Denial breeds misunderstanding. Your willingness to have open and honest discussions is vital. If you refuse to communicate (talk *and listen*), you are refusing to acknowledge and understand. If you refuse to acknowledge and understand, you are refusing to love. What could be more destructive to any relationship? By attempting to understand and support your loved one's struggle for freedom from diet/weight conflict, you (and she) can strengthen and enrich your lives in ways you would not have done otherwise.

ASSESSING YOUR PRESENT BEHAVIOR

The following behavior assessment can be used by anyone who wants to support health and well-being instead of diet/weight conflict and eating disorders. Use the following scale to indicate the frequency of each behavior listed below.

N = Never, R = Rarely, O = Occasionally, F = Frequently, D = Daily

HOW OFTEN DO YOU _____?:

Frequency

1. encourage someone* to pursue slenderness	N	R	O	F	D
2. encourage someone to "diet"	N	R	O	F	D
3. encourage someone to deprive herself of desired but "fattening" food	N	R	O	F	D
4. tease or admonish someone about her food or eating habits	N	R	O	F	D
5. criticize someone else's eating (habits or choices)	N	R	O	F	D
6. admire weight-loss diets or weight-loss dieting	N	R	O	F	D
7. admire rigidly controlled eating	N	R	O	F	D
8. criticize your own eating (habits or choices)	N	R	O	F	D
9. make negative comments about your fatness	N	R	O	F	D
10. make negative comments about someone else's fatness	N	R	O	F	D
11. directly or indirectly support the assumption that no one should be fat	N	R	O	F	D
12. disapprove of fatness (in general)	N	R	O	F	D

* "Someone" includes *anyone* (from a stranger to an immediate relative) except yourself.

13. say (or assume) that someone is "doing well" because she has lost weight	N	R	O	F	D
14. say something that presumes that a fat person (or people) wants to lose weight	N	R	O	F	D
15. say something that presumes that fat people should lose weight	N	R	O	F	D
16. say something that presumes that fat people eat too much	N	R	O	F	D
17. refer to "good" and "bad" food	N	R	O	F	D
18. talk about "being good" and "being bad" in reference to eating behavior	N	R	O	F	D
19. encourage someone to let go of guilt	N	R	O	F	D
20. encourage/approve of spontaneous eating	N	R	O	F	D
21. compliment someone's creativity	N	R	O	F	D
22. compliment someone's idea(s)	N	R	O	F	D
23. compliment someone's openness	N	R	O	F	D
24. compliment someone's efforts	N	R	O	F	D
25. compliment someone's sensitivity to others	N	R	O	F	D
26. say "I love you"	N	R	O	F	D
27. openly admire a fat person's appearance	N	R	O	F	D
28. openly admire a fat person	N	R	O	F	D
29. actively oppose fattism (verbally or in writing)	N	R	O	F	D
30. challenge myths about diet and weight	N	R	O	F	D
31. discourage self-criticism and competitiveness	N	R	O	F	D
32. encourage or admire self-acceptance and self-appreciation/love	N	R	O	F	D
33. talk about your appearance	N	R	O	F	D

For Sufferers' Loved Ones: Offering Support

34. talk about someone else's appearance	N	R	O	F	D
35. admire slenderness	N	R	O	F	D
36. talk about exercise for weight control/loss	N	R	O	F	D
37. admire obsessive exercise	N	R	O	F	D
38. talk about your weight	N	R	O	F	D
39. talk about someone else's weight	N	R	O	F	D
40. talk about calories	N	R	O	F	D
41. talk about how little you've eaten or your "diet"	N	R	O	F	D
42. encourage perfectionism	N	R	O	F	D
43. encourage conformity instead of self-determination and freedom	N	R	O	F	D
44. criticize someone	N	R	O	F	D

Making Your List of Personal Goals

Step A

Look at your answers for items 1–18. None of these actions is ever helpful. Therefore, for each item where you circled anything but N, you should set a personal goal to eliminate that (and similar) behavior. Make a list of personal goals on a piece of paper as you review your answers.

Step B

Look at your answers for items 19–32. All of these actions can be helpful. For each item where you circled N or R (for never or rarely), set a personal goal to increase that behavior. Add these goals to your list.

Step C

Look over your answers to items 33–44. These actions are usually unhelpful, but they do not call for an answer of N (for never). Answers of F or D (for frequently or daily) indicate a need for change. Read through the suggestions below for each item where you circled F or D, and add the needed goals to your list.

Corresponding Suggestions and Goals: Items 33–44

33 and 34. Talking about appearance is perfectly natural and acceptable; however, it is constantly done to excess. Our culture focuses on appearance (particularly women's appearance) far too much and objectifies people (partic-

ularly women), both of which encourage the development of diet/weight conflict and eating disorders. Counteractive measures are desperately needed.

The more you talk about appearance, the more you inflate its importance. We need to realize (and teach others) that appearance is much less important than health, happiness, character, and virtually every other human quality and concern. By refusing to focus on appearance, we can make a personal statement that it is a relatively minor concern. This will in turn promote the idea that the pursuit of physical "beauty" never merits self-destructive behavior.

35. Appreciating the physical beauty of slender people is fine, provided that you do not promote the idea that slenderness is a prerequisite for beauty. Appreciate the physical beauty of fat and "pudgy" people just as often, and don't forget to minimize *all* of these appearance-oriented comments.

36. Regular exercise is a great way to promote good health and well-being, but obsessive exercising for weight control is often a symptom of diet/weight conflict and eating disorders. Conversations that focus on exercise for weight loss and control are harmful because they rest on the assumption that we should try to eliminate body fat. If you want to talk about exercise, talk about it as a way to have fun and to feel good. Beware of talking about exercise (or the lack thereof) as anything

more than a personal choice. Our culture has inappropriately instilled exercise with moral implications. Remember that exercise increases people's physical fitness, *not* their personal value.

37. Admiring an athlete's training and accomplishment on occasion is one thing; admiring people's obsessive exercise programs is another. Beware of admiring obsessive exercise in general because your admiration will encourage people to cling to the weight conflict and eating disorders that are so often responsible for those exercise programs.

38 and 39. Discussions about weight can be positive if they refute popular myths or appreciate how helpful and healthy it has been for someone to stop dieting and maintain a comfortable, stable weight. People often need to talk about their weight as they struggle to make peace with their bodies and themselves. However, all the "usual" discussions about weight (which support popular myths and self-destructive behavior and goals) are harmful.

40. Sometimes it can be helpful to discuss myths about calories (for instance, the myth that 3,500 calories equals one pound of body fat when people overeat or undereat). However, discussions regarding the caloric content of foods are unnecessary, unhelpful, and often harmful. Only "dieters" worry and talk about calories. Don't encourage people to think and behave like dieters by having conversations about calories.

41. It's fine to make comments such as "I can't wait for dinner because I missed lunch." However, do not talk about restrictive diets, nor proudly announce that you haven't eaten much lately. Whenever you focus on meager eating as a personal triumph, need, or goal, you promote diet/weight conflict and eating disorders for yourself and the people around you.

42. Once in a long while we find a true need for perfection or near perfection, but in general, perfection is an unrealistic and destructive goal. People who suffer from diet/weight conflict and eating disorders are often (but not always) perfectionists, and perfectionism encourages their problem. Perfectionism requires a constant search for (and focus on) imperfections and faults. Encourage people to appreciate themselves and their accomplishments, however "imperfect" they may be.

43. If everyone constantly tried to conform to societal norms and expectations, the epidemic of eating disorders would be even worse than it is now. People need to make their own decisions and sort out their own values. Beware of *pushing* your own (or society's) values on other people, especially if the "other people" in question are your teenage children. (Teenagers have their own opinions. Offer your opinions and advice in a reasonable and respectful manner and they will be more likely to consider what you have to say.) Even when your intentions and "advice" are good, the effect of pressure is often harmful.

44. If you recognize a problem and a possible solution that another person does not seem to recognize, feel free to say so. However, stress your suggestion rather than your criticism. If you need to criticize, criticize choices or behavior rather than the person. Mix your constructive criticism with positive statements so that the person will know she is appreciated exactly as she is. Do not offer unconstructive criticism—it is not only unhelpful, but harmful.

Working on Your Goals

Now that you have defined your goals, you are ready to begin the hard work: changing your behavior. This has to be done moment by moment, as you catch yourself making destructive statements, for instance. Bravely admit your "slips" whenever you notice them, but don't be hard on yourself. It takes a lot of time and practice to change attitudes and habits you've formed over many years. Don't demand instant perfection from yourself because that would be unhelpful and unfair.

In order to keep progressing, review your goals very regularly. For the first two weeks, review them twice daily: once in the morning and once in the evening. This is especially important if you *live with* someone who is preoccupied with diet and weight. You and she have probably developed very destructive patterns that often go unnoticed. If you read your list of goals regularly and review your behavior carefully, you will soon see your errors.

You may also notice how your loved one(s) encourage your destructive comments and actions. Bravely point to these problems, but be sure to acknowledge the problems as destructive patterns you have created *together*. Placing "blame" is unhelpful. It truly does not matter who is more or less to blame. How you can effect change and thereby progress is what matters.

As you progress toward your goals, you can afford to review them less frequently. I recommend the following schedule:

Week 1–2: Twice daily review, first thing in the morning and last thing at night. Weekly reassessment of current behavior.

Week 3: One review every other day. Weekly reassessment of current behavior.

Weeks 4–8: One review each week. Weekly reassessment of current behavior.

Write your review schedule on a calendar or a piece of paper. Keep your schedule and list of goals in a readily accessible place. Try to review your goals at the same time of day and in the same place. This should help you stick to your schedule.

After your first two months of work, you will probably have made considerable progress, but your task will not be done. This is partly because you are constantly subjected to the same negative influences you are trying to stop supporting through your own words and actions. You may want to continue to review your goals on a regular basis in order to counteract all the insidious advertisements, conversations, etc. However, if you know your goals by heart and continually notice how you encourage and discourage diet/weight conflict, then you no longer need to reread them on a regular basis. In either case, good work! You have probably helped many people, some of whom you didn't even know were affected by your behavior.

RESOURCES: GETTING HELP AND RECOMMENDED READING

I wrote this book to help you let go of the diet/weight obsession, but *this book may not be enough for you*. If you are underweight, purging, very upset, or depressed, you need direct help through individual or group therapy. Feel free to use this book in *addition* to professional help, but don't use it in place of professional help.

During my senior year of college, my friend Sam noticed that I was going through hard times. He suggested that I go to the counseling center for help. My initial reaction was "Who me? You've got to be kidding!" However, I eventually realized that it was a good suggestion. My facade was cheerful and strong, but I knew that I wasn't nearly as happy as I pretended to be. Eventually, I took my friend's advice and benefited enormously.

Those of us who try to be independent have the hardest time getting help. We don't

trust anyone to help us. Getting help feels like a show of weakness. We want to do everything ourselves, without help from anyone. Realize here and now that getting help is *not* a sign of weakness or dependence. In fact, getting help is a show of strength. After all, in order to get help you must take the terrifying risk of acknowledging and working through the most painful issues in your life. Getting help is not a way of giving up on your ability to help yourself. Therapists don't "solve" their clients' problems nor tell them how to live. Therapists help their clients *help themselves*. Therefore, when you seek help you will be making a decision to reach out, open your eyes, explore, and work. You will be increasing your own efforts to grow.

Search your soul carefully: Do you hurt yourself? Do you isolate yourself? Are you hungry right now? Have you lost your periods? Are you fooling yourself about how you feel? Are you clinging to the edge of an emotional cliff? Have you shut out painful thoughts and feelings? Once you have answered these questions *honestly*, you'll be ready to decide whether or not you need professional counseling.

If you decide to see a therapist, choose carefully. Most therapists (like medical doctors) know very little about the human energy balance, nutrition, and eating disorders. Begin therapy on a trial basis. Do not work with a therapist who is openly fattist. If a therapist pressures you to lose weight, find someone else. If a therapist seems to feel that fat people are "too heavy" (unacceptable as they are), find someone else. Look for a therapist with a feminist/humanist orientation who will encourage you to make your own choices without being limited by cultural prescriptions.

Other concerns you should discuss with your therapist at the start of a new therapeutic relationship:

1. *Credentials:* is she/he licensed or in training for licensure in his/her field (usually social work, psychology, or psychiatry)?

2. *Experience:* does she/he have experience working with people who suffer from eating disorders and related problems?

3. *Cost:* what are his/her fees, and will treatment be covered by insurance? What is the usual billing procedure? Will you have to pay up front, before any insurance money comes through?

Ideally, you will want a licensed therapist who specializes, at least to some extent, in the treatment of eating disorders. Occasionally, one may find an experienced, effective therapist who lacks the usual credentials. In such a case, ask for a professional reference, follow up on that reference, and then rely on your own judgment. However, it is safer to select someone who is formally trained and licensed as well as experienced. These credentials will not guarantee an effective or ethical therapist, but they are a good start.

Most important, you will want a therapist with whom you feel comfortable. After a few sessions, be sure to ask yourself: "Do I trust this person? Do I feel able to be open and honest with him/her? Do I respect his/her attitude toward me and and toward my problems? Do I feel understood and not judged?" If the answer to any of these questions is no, discuss the way you feel with your therapist. Some feelings of discomfort and anxiety are normal at the start of therapy, but if you continue to feel uncomfortable after many more sessions, tell your therapist that you need a better "fit" and look for someone else. Remember: You need and deserve a therapist who fits your personality and needs. Do not feel guilty for ending therapy with someone who doesn't feel right.

Regardless of your body type, size, or eating disorder symptoms, you can benefit by letting go of your fattism and opposing it in your environment. One immediate way to move toward these goals is to learn about, and join, the National Association to Aid Fat Americans (NAAFA). This nonprofit organization is a *support group* for fat people and their admirers; an *educational organization* with newsletters, other mailings, and a "Fat Awareness" educational program; and a

---

human rights group that fights job discrimination, offensive advertising, lack of adequate and respectful health care, social discrimination, and related problems faced by fat people. The membership fee is nominal (special arrangements can be made for those with financial hardship), and all members receive the NAAFA newsletters. For more information about this progressive and important organization, write or call:

National Association to Aid Fat Americans
  P.O. Box 188620
  Sacramento, CA 95818
  (916) 443-0303

The following eating disorder associations can provide references to clinics, support groups, and therapists who specialize in eating disorders. (Even recommended therapists should be subjected to careful scrutiny.) *If your area lacks its own association, call the National Anorexic Aid Society in Ohio.* I strongly recommend that you call one of these associations *first.* In general, the people at these associations are extremely understanding, knowledgeable, and supportive. They can probably help you decide what to do next.

EATING DISORDER ASSOCIATIONS

National Anorexic Aid Society
  5796 Karl Road
  Columbus, OH 43229
  (614) 436-1112

Mental Health Association of Broward County
  2312 South Andrews Avenue
  Fort Lauderdale, FL 33316
  (305) 467-7766

ANAD—National Association of Anorexia Nervosa and Associated Disorders
  Box 7
  Highland Park, IL 60035
  (312) 831-3438
  (Individuals requesting information should send a self-addressed envelope with $.37 postage; organizations should send $1.00 to cover postage and handling.)

ABC—Anorexia, Bulimia Care, Inc.
  Box 213
  Lincoln Center, MA 01773
  (617) 259-9767

MAANA—Maryland Association for Anorexia Nervosa and Bulimia, Inc.
  P.O. Box 255
  Riderwood, MD 21139
  (301) 821-7378

American Anorexia/Bulimia Association, Inc.
  133 Cedar Lane
  Teaneck, NJ 07666
  (201) 836-1800

ANRED–Anorexia Nervosa and Related Eating Disorders, Inc.
  P.O. Box 5102
  Eugene, OR 97405
  (503) 344-1144

American Anorexia/Bulimia Association of Philadelphia, Inc.
  Philadelphia Child Guidance Clinic
  34th Street and Civic Center Boulevard
  Philadelphia, PA 19104
  (215) 244-2225

The following clinics and hospitals treat people suffering from eating disorders. This is not a comprehensive list of such services, but should include some in your region. Eating disorder clinics are springing up all over the country in response to the great need. For a more complete listing in your area, call your local eating disorder association or the National Anorexic Aid Society listed above.

IMPORTANT: Do *not* assume that the services listed here are in any way superior to any other eating disorder services. I am not recommending the services listed. Regardless of whether or not you use this listing, remember to subject your options to careful scrutiny.

EATING DISORDER CLINICS AND OTHER PROGRAMS— STATE BY STATE

Dr. James B. McLoong, Director
Eating Disorder Program
Institute of Behavioral Medicine
1111 East McDowell Road
Phoenix, AZ 85062
(602) 239–6880

Ginnie Grant Monroe, A.C.S.W.
Affiliated Counseling Service
7641 South 40th Place
Phoenix, AZ 85040
(602) 468–3850

Barton J. Blinder, M.D., Director
Eating Disorders Program
Department of Psychiatry and Human Behavior
College of Medicine
University of California at Irvine
Dana Point, CA 92629
(714) 831–6631

Rader Institute
Garden Grove Medical Center
12601 Garden Grove Boulevard
Garden Grove, CA 92643
(714) 537–5160, ext. 675

Frances Mead-Messinger, Ph.D., Executive Director
Sanivita Foundation, Inc.
16152 Beach Boulevard, Suite 180 East
Huntington Beach, CA 92647
(714) 842–0886

Rader Institute
North Hollywood Medical Center
12629 Riverside Drive
North Hollywood, CA 91607
(818) 766–9410

Mary Neal, Ph.D.
Eating Disorders Clinic
Neuropsychiatric Institute
Center for the Health Sciences
University of California at Los Angeles
760 Westwood Plaza
Los Angeles, CA 90024
(213) 825–8441 or –0271

Robbin I. Grossman, M.A., Program Director
Rader Institute
South Bay Hospital
514 North Prospect Avenue
Redondo Beach, CA 90277
(213) 318–4670 or –4702

Elaine Alexander, Program Director
Rader Institute/AMI
Mission Bay Hospital
3030 Bunker Hill Street
San Diego, CA 92109
(619) 274–7721, ext. 302
(619) 292–4885

Nancy T. Leenheer, D.M.H.
Mount Zion Eating Disorders Program
P.O. Box 7921
San Francisco, CA 94120
(415) 885–7415

Susan Owen, M.F.C.C., Program Director
  Eating Disorders Unit
  San Pedro Peninsula Hospital
  1300 West 7th Street, Annex B
  San Pedro, CA 90732
  (213) 514–5306

Bay Psychiatric Medical Group
  22503 Kent Ave., #A
  Torrance, CA 90505
  (213) 373–0527

Diane Green, Executive Director
  ADVANCE: Eating Disorders Treatment Program
  Memorial Hospital, Boulder
  Boulder, CO 80302
  (303) 441–0560
  (800) ADVANCE

Barbara E. Thomas, R.N., B.S.N.
  Eating Disorders Program
  Cedar Springs Hospital
  2135 Southgate Road
  Colorado Springs, CO 80906
  (719) 633–4114

The Rader Institute
  AMI/St. Luke's Hospital
  601 East 19th Avenue
  Denver, CO 80203
  (303) 869–2337
  (800) 255–1818

Dr. R. Timothy Pollak
  7345 South Pierce Street, Suite 201A
  Littleton, CO 80123
  (303) 972–0714

ADVANCE: Eating Disorders Treatment
  Fort Collins Outpatient
  Fort Collins, CO 80521
  (303) 484–6913
  (800) ADVANCE

Dr. Diane Mickley, Director
  Wilkins Center for Eating Disorders
  7 Riversville Road
  Greenwich, CT 06831
  (203) 531–1909

Dr. Bridberg/Mr. Hicky
  Institute of Living
  400 Retreat Avenue
  Hartford, CT 06102
  (203) 241–8000 or –6850

Geri French, M.S.W., Intake Coordinator
  Eating Disorder Service
  Newington Children's Hospital
  181 East Cedar Street
  Newington, CT 06111
  (203) 667–KIDS

Wheeler Clinic
  91 Northwest Drive
  Plainville, CT 06062
  (203) 747–6801

Dr. Richard Raborn, Medical Director
  Eating Disorders Program
  Bethesda Hospital
  2815 South Seacrest Boulevard
  Boynton Beach, FL 33435
  (407) 737–4300

Dr. Adrien Ressler, Director
  Eating Disorder Program
  Florida Medical Center
  5000 West Oakland Park Boulevard
  Fort Lauderdale, FL 33313
  (305) 735–6000, ext. 2411

Rader Institute
  North Ridge Medical Center
  5757 North Dixie Highway
  Fort Lauderdale, FL 33334
  (305) 776–6000, ext. 2138

Rader Institute
  Southeastern Medical Center
  1750 N.E. 167th Street
  North Miami Beach, FL 33162
  (305) 944–2550

Rader Institute
  Lake Seminole Hospital
  9675 Seminole Boulevard
  Seminole, FL 34642
  (813) 398–3350

Gerri Goodman, M.A., Program Coordinator
  Eating Disorders Program
  CPC Parkwood Hospital
  1999 Cliff Valley Way, N.E.
  Atlanta, GA 30329
  (404) 633–8431

Dr. Julio A. Molina, Director
  Anxiety Disorders Institute, Inc.
  1 Dunwoody Park, Suite 112
  Atlanta, GA 30338
  (404) 395–6845

Dr. Michael S. Barnett, Director
  Eating Disorders Program
  Intermountain Hospital
  303 Allumbaugh
  Boise, ID 83704
  (208) 377–8400

Chester Taranowski, A.C.S.W.
  Rader Institute
  Mount Sinai Hospital North
  2451 West Howard Street
  Chicago, IL 60645
  (312) 465–0995
  (312) 761–6000, ext. 5581

Regina Casper, M.D., Director
  Michael Reese Medical Center
  Psychosomatic and Psychiatric Institute
  Lake Shore Drive at 31st Street
  Chicago, IL 60616
  (312) 791–3957

Susan Sewell, Director
  Eating Disorders Program
  Swedish American Hospital
  1400 Charles Street
  Rockford, IL 61108
  (815) 968–4400

Brian J. Casey, Director
  BALANCE
  Winona Memorial Hospital
  3232 North Meridian Street
  Indianapolis, IN 46208
  (317) 927–2216

Sue J. Rhee, R.D.
  Eating Disorders Program
  Indiana University Hospitals
  926 West Michigan Street
  Indianapolis, IN 46223
  (317) 274–8928

Dr. Diane Alber
  Eating Disorders Program
  Mercy Hospital Medical Center
  Sixth and University
  Des Moines, IA 50314
  (515) 247–3192

Joyce Feddersen, R.N., M.A., Program Director
  Eating Disorders Unit
  Iowa Lutheran Hospital University at Penn
  Des Moines, IA 50316
  (515) 263–5258

Becky Reeves, M.S.W., Director
  Eating Disorders Program
  CPC Meadow Wood Hospital
  9032 Perkins Road
  Baton Rouge, LA 70810
  (504) 766–8553

Rader Institute
  Riverview Medical Center
  1125 West Louisiana Highway 30
  Gonzales, LA 70737
  (504) 647–5028

Marilyn Ackerman, Program Director
St. Jude Eating Disorder Center
180 West Esplanade
Kenner, LA 70065
(504) 464–8185

John Vance, B.C.S.W.
Eating Disorders Program
Coliseum Medical Center
3601 Coliseum
New Orleans, LA 70115
(504) 891–1401

Dr. Philip Lewandoski
McLean Hospital
Belmont, MA 02178
(617) 855–2000

David B. Herzog, M.D., Director
Eating Disorders Unit
Massachusetts General Hospital
55 Fruit Street
Boston, MA 02114
(617) 726–2724

Stanley Walzer, Ph.D., Director
Judge Baker Children's Center
295 Longwood Avenue
Boston, MA 02115
(617) 232–8390

George L. Blackburn, M.D., Ph.D.
Nutrition Coordinating Center
New England Deaconess Hospital
194 Pilgrim Road
Boston, MA 02215
(617) 732–8543 or –8544
(Outpatient treatment for adults only)

Blair Barone, M.A., Program Manager
Eating Disorder Program
Hahnemann Hospital
1515 Commonwealth Avenue
Brighton, MA 02135
(617) 254–1100, ext. 606

Laurie A. Silver, M.S.W.
Out-patient Eating Disorder Services
Neponset Valley Counseling Center
32 Baker Street
Foxboro, MA 02035
(617) 543–8888

Dr. Perry L. Belfer, Clinical Coordinator
The Eating Disorders Program
Newton-Wellesley Hospital
2014 Washington Street
Newton, MA 02162
(617) 243–6157

Teri Rumpf, Ph.D., Coordinator
Eating Disorders Program
University of Massachusetts Medical Center
55 Lake Avenue North
Worcester, MA 01655
(617) 739–7770
(617) 956–3220

Arnold E. Andersen, M.D., Director
Eating and Weight Disorders Clinic
Meyer Building, 3rd Floor, Room 181
Johns Hopkins Hospital
600 North Wolfe Street
Baltimore, MD 21205
(301) 955–3863

Dr. David Roth, Director
Eating Disorder Program
Sheppard-Pratt Hospital
6501 North Charles Street
Towson, MD 21204
(301) 337–6624

Nancy J. Shiller, M.A.C.P.
Race/Shiller Psychotherapists
31 Exchange Street
Portland, ME 04101
(207) 775–2833

David H. Vos, M.A., L.L.P., Director
Eating Disorders Program
Battle Creek Adventist Hospital
165 North Washington
Battle Creek, MI 49016
(800) 582–1900
(616) 964–7121, ext. 272

Antonino Cavaleri, Program Director
Holly Road Mental Health Center
8401 Holly Road
Grand Blanc, MI 48439
(313) 695–4600

Kathryn J. Miller, R.N., B.S.H.A., Program Manager
Pennant Eating Disorders Program
Saginaw General Hospital
1447 North Harrison
Saginaw, MI 48602
(517) 771–4855
(800) 642–0136

Richard L. Pyle, M.D., Director
Eating Disorder Program
University of Minnesota
Box 301, Mayo Memorial Building
420 Delaware Street, S.E.
Minneapolis, MN 55455
(612) 626–6188

Richard Justman, M.A., Medical Director
The Institute for Eating Disorders
Methodist Hospital
6500 Excelsior Boulevard
St. Louis Park, MN 55440
(612) 932–6200

Ann S. Gabrick, L.S.C.S.W., Program Manager
Eating Disorders Program
Menorah Medical Center
4949 Rockhill Road
Kansas City, MO 64110
(816) 276–8486

Nancy Ellis-Ordway, A.C.S.W., Contact Person
Anorexia Bulimia Treatment and Education Center
St. John's Mercy Medical Center
615 South New Ballas, Suite 7019-B
St. Louis, MO 63141
(314) 569–6898
(800) 222–2832

John W. Sanders, Education and Training
Eating Disorders Program
St. Anthony's Medical Center
10016 Kennerly Road
St. Louis, MO 63128
(314) 525–1800

Felix E. Larocca, M.D.
BASH—Bulimia, Anorexia, Self-Help
Suite 215, 6125 Clayton Avenue
St. Louis, MO 63139
(314) 567–4080

Rader Institute
Springfield Community Hospital
3535 South National Avenue
Springfield, MO 65807
(417) 882–6950

Robert Lynn Horne, M.D., Director
Eating Disorders Program
HCA Montevista Center
6000 West Rochelle Avenue, #700
Las Vegas, NV 89102
(702) 364–1177

Dr. Wilfred Postel, Director
Eating Disorders Program
Carrier Foundation
P.O. Box 147
Belle Mead, NJ 08502
(201) 874–4000

Linnea Lindholm, Project Coordinator
Rutgers Eating Disorders Clinic
Piscataway, NJ 08854
(201) 932–2292

Karen M. McLeod, B.S.N., R.N.
  Fair Oaks Hospital
  19 Prospect Street
  Summit, NJ 07901
  (201) 522–7035

Linda Cumberland, Director
  Anorexia-Bulimia Treatment Program
  Kaseman Presbyterian Hospital
  8300 Constitution, N.E.
  Albuquerque, NM 87110
  (505) 291–2506

Craig House Hospital
  Howland Avenue
  Beacon, NY 12508
  (312) 831–3438

Mary Anne Cohen, C.S.W., Director
  The New York Center for Eating Disorders
  490 Third Street
  Brooklyn, NY 11215
  (718) 788–6986

Dr. Melanie Katzman, Clinical Director
  Psychiatric Outpatient Services
  Regent Hospital
  425 East 61st Street
  New York, NY 10016
  (212) 935–3400 .

B. Timothy Walsh, M.D., Director
  Eating Disorders Research and Treatment Program
  New York State Psychiatric Institute
  Columbia Presbyterian Medical Center
  722 West 168th Street
  New York, NY 10032
  (212) 960–5752 or –5754

William Davis, Ph.D., Executive Director
  Center for the Study of Anorexia and Bulimia
  1 West 91st Street
  New York, NY 10024
  (212) 595–3449

William Owen, M.D.
  Eating Disorders Program
  Stony Lodge Hospital
  Croton Dam Road
  Ossining, NY 10510
  (914) 941–7400, ext. 225

Katherine A. Halmi, M.D., Director
  Eating Disorders Program
  New York Hospital–Cornell Medical Center
  Westchester Division
  21 Bloomingdale Road
  White Plains, NY 10605
  (914) 997–5875

Jerald Lane, M.D., Medical Director
  Eating Disorders Program
  Charter Pines Hospital
  3621 Randolph Road
  Charlotte, NC 28211
  (704) 365–5368

Dr. Robin N. Moir, Director
  Eating Disorders Center of Cleveland
  St. Vincent Medical Building, Suite 302
  2322 East 22nd Street
  Cleveland, OH 44115
  (216) 363–2780

Dr. David Lombard
  Eating Disorders, Department of Psychiatry
  Kettering Medical Center
  3535 Southern Boulevard
  Kettering, OH 45429
  (513) 296–7827

Kay L. Grothaus, M.S.W., C.S., Director
  Eating Disorders Program
  St. Vincent Medical Center
  2213 Cherry Street
  Toledo, OH 43608
  (419) 255–5665

Mary Ann O'Loughlin, M.S., L.P.C., Program Director
Rader Institute
Southwestern Medical Center
5602 West Lee Boulevard
Lawton, OK 73505
(405) 531-4722

Billie Hunter, Program Manager
Eating Disorders Unit
Hillcrest Medical Center
1120 South Utica
Tulsa, OK 74104
(918) 560-5711

Veronica Jeffus, M.Ed., L.P.C., Director
Rader Institute
Doctor's Hospital
2323 South Harvard
Tulsa, OK 74114
(918) 742-1081

Dr. Jean Rubel, Director
Eating Disorders Program
Sacred Heart Hospital
1255 Hilyard Street
Eugene, OR 97401
(503) 344-1144

Brenda Hickethier, Administrative Director
ADVANCE: Eating Disorders Treatment Program
Portland Adventist Medical Center
10123 S.E. Market Street
Portland, OR 97229
(503) 251-6101

Sandra Kelly, R.D., Outpatient Services Director
Eating Disorders Program
CPC Cedar Hills Hospital
10300 S.W. Eastridge Street
Portland, OR 97225
(503) 297-2252

Jeri C. Graham, R.C.S.W.
Private Professional Counseling
433 S.E. Main
Roseburg, OR 97470
(503) 673-8404

Sandra McCarthy, R.N., Clinical Supervisor
Tri-State Eating Disorders Center
The Medical Center
1000 Dutch Ridge Road
Beaver, PA 15009
in PA: (800) 622-2832
outside: (800) 782-2832

Dr. Neal R. Satten, Director
The Institute of Pennsylvania Hospital
111 North 49th Street
Philadelphia, PA 19139
(215) 471-2384

Dr. Leonard S. Levitz, Clinical Director
Dr. Joan E. Enoch, Medical Director
The Renfrew Center
475 Spring Lane
Philadelphia, PA 19128
(215) 482-5353
(800) 334-8415

Dr. Susan Ice, Director
Eating Disorders Program
Philadelphia Psychiatric Center
Ford and Monument Avenue
Philadelphia, PA 19131
(215) 581-5489

Debby Hay, Coordinator
Eating Disorder Program
Warminster Hospital
225 Newtown Road
Warminster, PA 18974
(215) 441-6900

Cathy D. Killian, Program Director
Rader Institute
Piedmont Medical Center
222 South Herlong Avenue
Rock Hill, SC 29730
(803) 329-6864

Resources: Getting Help and Recommended Reading

Rader Institute
  Frye Regional Medical Center
  420 North Center Street
  Hickory, SC 28601
  (704) 324–3450

Elizabeth Moody, Program Director
  Eating Disorders Program
  Methodist Central
  1265 Union Avenue
  Memphis, TN 38104
  (901) 726–7878

Maribeth Flood, R.N., M.S., Program Coordinator
  Eating Disorder Unit
  CPC Millwood Hospital
  1011 North Cooper Street
  Arlington, TX 76011
  (817) 261–3121, ext. 330

Jana Russell, Director
  Eating Disorders Program
  St. David's Community Hospital
  Austin, TX 78705
  (512) 397–4023

Martha Collier, CADAC
  New Spirit
  Texas Woman's Hospital
  7600 Fanin
  Houston, TX 77054
  (713) 790–1234, ext. 5999

Dr. Davis Krueger, Medical Director
  Eating Disorders Program
  Spring Shadow Glen
  2801 Gessner
  Houston, TX 77080
  (713) 462–4000

Beth Roseland, Director
  Eating Disorders Program
  Huguley Memorial Hospital
  11801 South Freeway
  Ft. Worth, TX 76123
  (817) 551–2788

Anne Turner, Program Manager
  CareUnit Hospital
  1066 West Magnolia
  Ft. Worth, TX 76104
  (817) 336–2828

Rader Institute
  North Texas Medical Center
  1800 North Graves Street
  McKinney, TX 75069
  (214) 548–3030

Mona Carey, L.C.S.W., M.A.S., Program Director
  Eating Disorders Program
  2960 Sleepy Hollow Road
  Falls Church, VA 22044
  (703) 536–2000

Randolyn Halterman, Program Manager
  Eating Disorders Center of Virginia
  Sentara Norfolk General Hospital
  600 Gresham Drive
  Norfolk, VA 23507
  (804) 628–2027

Dr. Maria Urbano, Director
  Women's Treatment Center
  Psychiatric Institute of the Medical College of
  Hampton Roads
  721 Fairfax Avenue
  Norfolk, VA 23507
  (804) 446–5180

Brattleboro Retreat
  Brattleboro, VT 05301
  (802) 257–7785
  (800) 345–5550

Dr. Michael D. Nugent, Program Administrator
  Rader Institute
  Auburn General Hospital
  20 Second Street, N.E.
  Auburn, WA 98002
  (206) 833–6508

Dr. Steve Stephenson, *Program Director*
Rader Institute
Riverton Hospital
12844 Military Road South
Seattle, WA 98168
(206) 248–4504

Kathleen Campbell, Program Director
Eating Disorders Unit
Ballard Community Hospital
N.W. Market and Barnes
Seattle, WA 98107
(206) 789–9345

Shane Thompson
Eating Disorders Program
St. Mary's Hospital
2900 First Avenue
Huntington, WV 25701
(304) 526–1570

Dr. Anthony T. Machi, Medical Director
Eating Disorders Program
St. Mary's Hill Hospital
2350 North Lake Drive
Milwaukee, WI 53211
(414) 271–5555

Eating Disorders Program
Pine Ridge Hospital
150 Wyoming
Lander, WY 82520
(307) 332–5700
(800) 922–5700

If you are interested in Overeaters Anonymous, check your local telephone directory. If it's not listed, write or call:

Overeaters Anonymous Headquarters
World Service Office
P.O. Box 92870
Los Angeles, CA 90009
(213) 542–8363

RECOMMENDED READING

We all know about "suggested" reading lists. Those are the widely ignored lists that often appear in books and course syllabi. Schools have taught many of us to dread reading. We have been forced to study so many topics we found uninteresting, and we have been forced to parrot so many teachers' viewpoints (instead of creating and exploring our own), that we may associate reading, and even learning, with boredom and frustration.

If you are one of the many who have been turned off from reading and learning, turn yourself back on. Make the time to learn about something that really interests you, knowing that what you learn can change you and your life for the better. Leo Buscaglia writes, "You know, learning is the greatest joy. To learn something is fantastic because every time you learn something you become something new."[1]

The following list focuses on books and articles that you, as a person who suffers from diet/weight conflict, might be interested in. However, it is *not* a comprehensive list of books about diet/weight conflict and eating disorders—very far from it. I do not recommend that you study eating disorders because that will not help you let go of your preoccupation, and it could have the opposite effect. (In fact, my first two years of research intensified my preoccupation. I had to take a break from the subject in order to let go of it.) Instead, focus on learning how to be assertive, how to build satisfying relationships, how to break free from fattism, and how to become a more actively loving person.

About Loving

Buscaglia, Leo. *Love*. Thorofare, N.J.: Slack, 1972.

Buscaglia, Leo. *Loving Each Other: The Challenge of Human Relationships.* Thorofare, N.J.: Slack, 1984.

Jampolsky, Gerald. *Love Is Letting Go of Fear.* N.Y.: Bantam, 1970.

Un-Learning Fattism

Ansfield, Alice, ed. *Radiance* Magazine. To subscribe, send $10 (one year: four issues) to: Radiance, P.O. Box 31703, Oakland, CA 94604–9937.

Bennett, William, M.D., and Gurin, Joel. *The Dieter's Dilemma: Eating Less and Weighing More.* N.Y.: Basic Books, 1982.

Chernin, Kim. *The Obsession: Reflections on the Tyranny of Slenderness.* N.Y.: Harper & Row, 1981.

Ernsberger, Paul, and Haskew, Paul. *Rethinking Obesity: An Alternative View of Its Health Implications.* N.Y.: Human Sciences Press, 1987.*

Grosswirth, Marvin. *Fat Pride: A Survival Handbook.* N.Y.: Jarrow Press, 1971.*

Louderback, Llewellyn. *Fat Power: Whatever You Weigh Is Right.* N.Y.: Hawthorn, 1970.*

National Association to Aid Fat Americans (NAAFA) Monthly Newsletters. Write to: NAAFA, P.O. Box 188620, Sacramento, CA 95818. Or call: (916) 443–0303.

* This book can be difficult to find; however, it is available by mail from the NAAFA Book Service (see address and phone number above).

Relearning Complete Sexual Satisfaction

Barbach, Lonnie. *For Yourself.* N.Y.: Doubleday, 1975.

Barbach, Lonnie. *For Each Other*. N.Y.: Anchor Press/Doubleday, 1982.

Blank, Joani. *The Play Book for Women About Sex*. Burlingame, Calif.: Down There Press, 1975.†

Blank, Joani. *The Play Book for Men About Sex*. Burlingame, Calif.: Down There Press, 1976.

Blank, Joani. *Good Vibrations: The Complete Women's Guide to Vibrators*. Burlingame, Calif.: Down There Press, 1982.

Dodson, Betty. *Selflove and Orgasm*. N.Y.: Betty Dodson, 1983. Republished with *Liberating Masturbation* as *Sex for One: The Joy of Selfloving*. N.Y.: Crown, 1987.

† For order information on Joani Blank's books, write to: Down There Press, P.O. Box 2086, Burlingame, CA 94010.

About Anorexia, Bulimia, and Compulsive Eating*

Hall, Lindsey, and Cohn, Leigh. *Bulimia: A Guide to Recovery*. Carlsbad, Calif.: Gurze Books, 1986.

Haskew, Paul, and Adams, Cynthia. *When Food Is a Four-Letter Word*. Englewood Cliffs, N.J.: Prentice-Hall, 1984.

Roth, Geneen. *Breaking Free from Compulsive Eating*. N.Y.: Bobbs-Merrill, 1984.

Sandbek, Terence J. *The Deadly Diet: Recovering from Anorexia and Bulimia*. Oakland, Calif.: New Harbinger, 1986.

Siegel, Michele; Brisman, Judith; and Weinshel, Margot. *Surviving an Eating Disorder: New Perspectives and Strategies for Family and Friends*. N.Y.: Harper & Row, 1988.

* For a free mail-order catalog of books on eating disorders, send your request for the "Eating Disorders Bookshelf Catalog—MPF" to: Gurze Books, P.O. Box 2238, Carlsbad, CA 92008.

Improving Body Image

The Boston Women's Health Book Collective. *The New Our Bodies, Ourselves* (3rd ed.). N.Y.: Simon and Schuster, 1984.

Hutchinson, Marcia Germaine. *Transforming Body Image*. Trumansburg, N.Y.: Crossing Press, 1985.

Rush, Anne Kent. *Getting Clear*. N.Y.: Random House, 1973; Berkeley, Calif.: The Bookworks, 1973.

Healthy Cookbooks

Allen, Francine. *Eating Well in a Busy World*. Berkeley, Calif.: Ten Speed Press, 1986.

Brody, Jane. *Good Food Book: Living the High-Carbohydrate Way*. N.Y.: Norton, 1985.

Burros, Marian. *Keep It Simple*. N.Y.: Pocket Books, 1981.

Gaunt, La Rene. *Recipes to Lower Your Fat Thermostat*. Provo, Utah: Vitality House International, 1984.

Leonard, Jon, and Taylor, Elaine. *The Live Longer Now Cookbook*. N.Y.: Grosset and Dunlap, 1977.

Robertson, Laurel; Flinders, Carol; and Ruppenthal, Brian. *The New Laurel's Kitchen*. Berkeley, Calif.: Ten Speed Press, 1986.

About Nutrition

Ballentine, Rudolph, M.D. *Diet and Nutrition: A Wholistic Approach* (2nd ed.). Honesdale, Penn.: Himalayan International Institute, 1984.

Brody, Jane. *Jane Brody's Nutrition Book*. N.Y.: Bantam, 1987.

Dye-Gossow, Joan, and Thomas, Paul R. *The Nutrition Debate: Sorting Out Some Answers*. Palo Alto, Calif.: Bull Publishing, 1987.

Leonard, Jon; Pritikin, Nathaniel; and Hoffer, Jack. *Live Longer Now*. N.Y.: Grosset and Dunlap, 1974.

Other Books of Interest

Bass, Ellen, and Davis, Laura. *The Courage to Heal: A Guide for Women Survivors of Child Sexual Abuse.* N.Y.: Harper & Row, 1988.

Biffle, Christopher. *The Castle of the Pearl.* (A guided journal of self-discovery.) N.Y.: Barnes and Noble, 1983.

Bloom, Lynn; Coburn, Karen; and Pearlman, Joan. *The New Assertive Woman.* (A woman's guide to becoming more assertive.) N.Y.: Dell, 1975.

Bolles, Richard. *What Color Is Your Parachute?* (rev. ed.). (A guide for career exploration.) Berkeley, Calif.: Ten Speed Press, 1982.

Branden, Nathaniel. *Breaking Free* (A guide for exploring and letting go of harmful messages you have received about yourself.) N.Y.: Bantam, 1970.

Dowling, Colette. *The Cinderella Complex: Women's Hidden Fear of Independence.* N.Y.: Simon and Schuster, 1981.

Steffen, James, and Steffen, Erika. *How Outstanding People Manage Time.* (A guide to better time management; comes with a special date/time organizer.) Stamford, Conn.: Steffen, Steffen and Associates, 1979.*

* For order information, write to: 652 Glenbrook Road, Stamford, CT 06906. Or call: (203) 359–4100.

NOTES

CHAPTER 1

1. Paul Ernsberger, "The Death of Dieting," *American Health* (January–February, 1985), pp. 29–33.

Ernsberger, "Neuralmediation of Genetic and Nutritional Effects on Blood Pressure," Ph.D. diss., Northwestern University, 1985.

2. Kim Chernin, *The Obsession: Reflections on the Tyranny of Slenderness* (N.Y.: Harper & Row, 1981).

3. This book was originally intended as a self-help program for *anyone* who is troubled by diet and weight; hence, most of its content can be helpful to men as well as women. However, much of Chapter 3 and the first part of Chapter 6 (the text, not the personal questions) focus exclusively on female sufferers' experiences and needs.

4. K. Halmi, J. Falk, and E. Schwartz, "Binge-Eating and Vomiting: A Survey of a College Population," *Psychological Medicine* (November 1981), 11(4):697–706.

H. G. Pope, J. I. Hudson, D. Yurgelon-Todd, and M. S. Hudson, "Prevalence of Anorexia Nervosa and Bulimia in Three Student Populations," *International Journal of Eating Disorders* (1984), 3:45–53.

CHAPTER 2

1. William Bennett, M.D., and Joel Gurin, *The Dieter's Dilemma: Eating Less and Weighing More* (N.Y.: Basic Books, 1982).

2. J. S. Garrow, *Energy Balance and Obesity in Man* (N.Y.: American Elsevier, 1974).

3. R. L. Goldman, "The Effects of the Manipulation of the Visibility of Food on the Eating Behavior of Obese and Normal Subjects," Ph.D. diss., Columbia University, 1968.

M. J. Mahoney, "The Obese Style: Bites, Beliefs, and Behavior Modification," *Addictive Behaviors* (1975), 1:47–53.

P. Pliner and G. Iuppa, "Effects of Increasing Awareness on Food Consumption in Obese and Normal Weight Subjects," *Addictive Behaviors* (1978), 3(1):19–24.

A. Stunkard, "Eating Patterns and Obesity," *Psychiatric Quarterly* (1959), 33:284.

4. C. P. Herman and D. Mack, "Restrained and Unrestrained Eating," *Journal of Personality* (1975), pp. 646–660.

C. P. Herman and J. Polivy, "Anxiety, Restraint, and Eating Behavior," *Journal of Abnormal Psychology* (1975), 84:666–672.

J. Spencer and W. J. Fremouw, "Binge Eating as a Function of Restraint and Weight Classification," *Journal of Abnormal Psychology* (June 1979), 88(3):262–267.

5. Six additional studies cited by S. C. Wooley, O. W. Wooley, and S. Dyrenforth, "Theoretical, Practical, and Social Issues in Behavioral Treatments of Obesity," *Journal of Applied Behavior Analysis* (Spring 1979), 12(1):3–25.

6. H. A. Guthrie, *Introductory Nutrition*, 4th ed. (St. Louis, Mo.: C. V. Mosby, 1979).

7. Basal metabolism rises during adolescence as a result of physical development. After full adult size has been reached, metabolism gradually decreases by approximately 35 calories/day (total) between ages 25 and 35, and 145 calories/day between ages 35 and 55. Thus individual adult metabolic rates decrease slightly with age. Body size directly correlates with metabolic rate: the taller and more massive the individual, the higher metabolism is likely to be. Body composition influences metabolism because muscle tissue requires more energy for maintenance than fat; consequently, those with greater amounts of muscle tend to have higher metabolisms.

In light of the above information, it is not surprising that gender is considered a determining factor of metabolism. On the average, men's metabolisms are higher than women's. Sex differences in metabolism appear to be especially strong between young men and women (approximately 17 to 20 years old). Young men often have very high metabolisms, while most young women do not.

8. P. M. Warwick, R. Toft, and J. S. Garrow, *Recent Advances in Obesity Research II: Proceedings of the International Congress on Obesity* (London: Newman, 1978).

9. G. A. Rose and R. T. Williams, "Metabolic Studies on Large and Small Eaters," *British Journal of Nutrition* (1961), 15:1.

10. Garrow, *Energy Balance.*

11. R. Mahler, "The Relationship Between Eating and Obesity," *Acta Diabetologica Latina 9*, Suppl. 1 (1972), p. 449.

12. Garrow, *Energy Balance.*

13. Wooley, Wooley, and Dyrenforth, "Behavioral Treatments of Obesity."

14. D. Miller and P. Mumford, "Gluttony: Thermogenesis in Overeating Man," *American Journal of Clinical Nutrition* (1967), 20: 1223–1229.

15. M. Apfelbaum, J. Bostsarron, and D. Lactis, "Effect of Caloric Restriction and Excessive Caloric Intake on Energy Expenditure," *American Journal of Clinical Nutrition* (1971), 24:1405.

16. Garrow, *Energy Balance.*

17. Paul Ernsberger, "The Death of Dieting," *American Health* (January–February 1985), pp. 29–33.

18. Consensus Development Conference, 1985, "Health Implications of Obesity," *Annals of Internal Medicine*, 103:1073–1077.

19. Paul Ernsberger and Paul Haskew, *Rethinking Obesity: An Alternative View of Its Health Implications* (N.Y.: Human Sciences Press, 1987), p. 18.

20. Ibid., p. 6.

21. Ibid., p. 36.

22. Consensus Development Conference, 1985.

23. Ernsberger, "The Death of Dieting."

24. Kim Chernin, *The Obsession: Reflections on the Tyranny of Slenderness* (N.Y.: Harper & Row, 1981).

25. Ernsberger and Haskew, *Rethinking Obesity*, p. 35.

26. Ibid., p. 10.

27. Jean Mayer, *Obesity: Causes, Costs, and Control* (Englewood Cliffs, N.J.: Prentice-Hall, 1968).

28. Peter Dally and Joan Gomez, *Obesity and Anorexia Nervosa: A Question of Shape* (London: Faber and Faber, 1980).

29. Mayer, *Obesity*, pp. 53–54 (describes a 1937 study by Newman).

30. Ancel Keys, J. Brosek, A. Henschel, A. Meckelsen, and H. L. Taylor, *The Biology of Human Star-*

vation (Minneapolis, Minn.: University of Minnesota Press, 1950).

31. M. L. Gluckman, J. Hirsch, R. S. McCully, B. A. Brown, and J. L. Knittle, "The Response of Obese Patients to Weight Reduction: A Quantitative Evaluation of Behavior," *Psychosomatic Medicine* (1968), 30:359–373.

32. Hilde Bruch, *Eating Disorders: Obesity, Anorexia Nervosa, and the Person Within* (N.Y.: Basic Books, 1973).

33. Garrow, *Energy Balance.*

34. Dennis Remington, M.D., Garth Fisher, and Edward Parent, *How to Lower Your Fat Thermostat* (Provo, Utah: Vitality House International, 1983).

35. Reubin Andres, M.D., Edwin L. Bierman, M.D., and William R. Hazzard, M.D., *Principles of Geriatric Medicine* (N.Y.: McGraw-Hill, 1984), pp. 311–318.

36. B. Guy-Grand and Y. Sitt, "Gustative Aliesthesia: Evidence Supporting the Ponderostatic Hypothesis for Obesity," in A. Howard (ed.), *Recent Advances in Obesity Research* (London: Newman, 1975), 1:238–241.

37 and 38. J. Wurtman, R. Wurtman, J. Growdon, P. Henry, A. Lipscomb, and S. Zeisel, "Carbohydrate Craving in Obese People: Suppression by Treatments Affecting Serotoninergic Transmission," *International Journal of Eating Disorders* (Autumn 1981).

CHAPTER 3

1. S. Jourard and P. Secord, "Body-Cathexis and the Ideal Female Figure," *Journal of Abnormal and Social Psychology* (1955), 33:625–629.

I conducted a more recent study (1980) at Wesleyan University. When I asked a random sample of twenty-five women to specify their "ideal weights," five gave weights well below the lowest recommended weights for their heights, and ten specified the lowest recommended weights (plus or minus one pound). Only seven women specified ideal weights that fell within the medium-frame ranges, and of these seven, five felt that they had given up their aesthetic ideals for more easily maintained and comfortable weights. (The remaining woman did not want to specify an ideal weight.) Not one woman I interviewed specified an ideal weight that fell into the range of recommended weights for large frames.

Male college undergraduates did not tend to choose the lowest recommended weights for their heights. Their personal ideals varied widely and fairly evenly around the mean of the standard recommended weights for medium frames. Some men's personal ideals fell within the standard ranges for small frames; others' fell within the medium- or large-frame ranges. Not one male undergraduate specified a personal ideal below the lowest recommended weight for his height.

2. E. Clifford, "Body Satisfaction in Adolescence," *Perceptual and Motor Skills* (1971), 33:119–125.

H. I. Douty, J. B. Moore, and D. Hartford, "Body Characteristics in Relation to Life Adjustment, Body-Image, and Attitudes of College Females," *Perceptual and Motor Skills* (1974), 39:499–521.

Llewelyn Louderback, *Fat Power* (N.Y.: Hawthorn, 1970).

3. Hilde Bruch, *Eating Disorders: Obesity, Anorexia Nervosa, and the Person Within* (N.Y.: Basic Books, 1973).

4. Marcia Millman, *Such a Pretty Face* (N.Y.: Norton, 1980).

5. Bruch, *Eating Disorders.*

6. Kim Chernin, *The Obsession: Reflections on the Tyranny of Slenderness* (N.Y.: Harper & Row, 1981).

7. Ken Smith, *Flower of Gold* (N.Y.: Tower Publications, 1982).

8. All names used in the text of this book have been changed.

9. George Lucas, *The Empire Strikes Back* (Los Angeles, Calif.: Lucasfilms, 1980).

10. Louderback, *Fat Power.*

11. J. R. Staffieri, "A Study of Social Stereotype of Body Image in Children," *Journal of Personality and Social Psychology* (1967), 7:101–104.

Staffieri, "Body Build and Behavioral Expectancies in Young Females," *Developmental Psychology* (1972), 6:125–127.

12. H. Canning and J. Mayer, "Obesity—Its Possible Effect on College Acceptance," *New England Journal of Medicine* (1966), 275:1172–1174.

13. Louderback, *Fat Power*.

14. For a list of the American Youth Hostel Offices ("Councils"), write to: American Youth Hostels, National Administrative Offices, 1332 "I" Street, N.W., Washington, DC 20005.

CHAPTER 4

1. Hilde Bruch, *Eating Disorders: Obesity, Anorexia Nervosa, and the Person Within* (N.Y.: Basic Books, 1973).

2. Robert Atkins, *Dr. Atkins' Diet Revolution: The High-Calorie Way to Stay Thin Forever* (N.Y.: David McKay, 1972).

3. Jon Leonard, Nathaniel Pritikin, and Jack Hoffer, *Live Longer Now* (N.Y.: Grosset and Dunlap, 1974).

4. Judy Manzel, *The Beverly Hills Diet* (N.Y.: Berkley, 1981).

5. E. M. Berman, "Factors Influencing Motivations in Dieting," *Journal of Nutrition Education* (October–December 1975), vol. 7, no. 4.

6. Susie Orbach, *Fat Is a Feminist Issue* (N.Y.: Berkley, 1978). Many of the women Orbach has worked with, as well as people with whom I have worked, serve as examples.

7. Frank Herbert, *Dune* (N.Y.: Berkley, 1965).

CHAPTER 5

1. Nathaniel Branden, *The Psychology of Self-Esteem: A New Concept of Man's Psychological Nature* (N.Y.: Bantam, 1969).

2. Susie Orbach, *Fat Is a Feminist Issue* (N.Y.: Berkley, 1978).

3. Gerald Jampolsky, *Love Is Letting Go of Fear* (N.Y.: Bantam, 1982).

4. Loosely modeled after "Litany Against Fear" in Frank Herbert's *Dune* (N.Y.: Berkley, 1965).

5. Zig Ziglar, *See You at the Top* (Gretna, La: Pelican, 1975).

6. Jampolsky, *Love Is Letting Go of Fear*.

7. Timothy Gallwey, *The Inner Game of Tennis* (N.Y.: Random House, 1974).

CHAPTER 6

1. M. Wittig and A. Petersen (eds.), *Sex-Related Differences in Cognitive Functioning* (N.Y.: Academic Press, 1979).

2. J. Veroff, S. Wilcox, and J. Atkinson, "The Achievement Motive in High School and College Women," *Journal of Abnormal Psychology* (1953), 48:108–119.

E. French and G. Lesser, "Some Characteristics of Achievement Motive in Women," *Journal of Abnormal Social Psychology* (1964), 68:2.

M. Mednick and P. Weston, "Race, Social Class, and the Motive to Avoid Success in Women," in J. M. Bardwick (ed.), *Readings on the Psychology of Women* (N.Y.: Harper & Row, 1972), pp. 68–71.

M. Horner, "Toward an Understanding of Achievement Related Conflicts in Women," *Journal of Social Issues* (1972), 28:157–175.

3. I. Broverman, D. Broverman, F. Clarkson, P. Rosenkratz, and S. Vogel, "Sex-Role Stereotypes and Clinical Judgements of Mental Health," in Bardwick (ed.), *Readings on the Psychology of Women* (N.Y.: Harper & Row, 1972).

4. Colette Dowling, *The Cinderella Complex* (N.Y.: Simon and Schuster, 1981).

5. Broverman et al., "Sex-Role Stereotypes."

6. S. L. Bem, "The Measurement of Psychological Androgyny," *Journal of Consulting and Clinical Psychology* (1974), 42:155–162.

Bem, "Sex-Role Adaptability: One Consequence of Psychological Androgyny," *Journal of Personality and Social Psychology* (1975), 31:634–643.

J. Spence and R. Helreich, *Masculinity and Femininity: Their Psychological Dimension, Correlates, and Antecedents* (Austin, Tex.: University of Texas Press, 1978).

7. A phrase Edith Berman used (paraphrasing Hilde Bruch) in a personal interview regarding common reactions to weight loss. Mrs. Berman was one of the originators of a well-known chain of weight-loss clinics. She has designed, researched, and led many weight-loss groups and has published a book and journal articles within this field.

8. James and Erika Steffen, *How Outstanding People Manage Time* (Stamford, Conn.: Steffen, Steffen and Associates, 1979).

9. Fred Small, "Everything Possible" (Pine Barrens Music [BMI], 1983). "Everything Possible" is recorded on Fred Small's album "No Limit" (Rounder Records, 1 Camp Street, Cambridge, MA 02140).

CHAPTER 8

1. H. A. Guthrie, *Introductory Nutrition*, 4th ed. (St. Louis, Mo: C.V. Mosby, 1979).

2. William Dufty, *Sugar Blues* (Radnor, Penn.: Chilton, 1975).

3. S. Turner and G. Mayer, "How to Read Between the Lines of Label Claims," *Nutrition Action* (October 1981), pp. 9–11.

4. Jon Leonard, Nathaniel Pritikin, and Jack Hoffer, *Live Longer Now* (N.Y.: Grosset and Dunlap, 1974).

5. United States Department of Agriculture, National Food Review-13 (Winter 1981).

6. Jane Brody, *Good Food Book: Living the High-Carbohydrate Way* (N.Y.: Norton, 1985), p. 19.

7. Ibid., p. 20.

8. Ibid., p. 18.

9. Joan Dye-Gossow and Paul R. Thomas, *The Nutrition Debate: Sorting Out Some Answers* (Palo Alto, Calif.: Bull Publishing, 1987).

10. Jane Brody, *Jane Brody's Nutrition Book* (N.Y.: Bantam, 1987), p. 444.

11. Dennis W. Remington, M.D., and Barbara W. Higa, *The Bitter Truth About Artificial Sweeteners* (Provo, Utah: Vitality House International, 1987).

12. Bonnie Liebman and the authors of "Nutrition Action," *Smart Eating Guide* (Washington, D.C.: Center for Science in the Public Interest, 1984).

13. Center for Science in the Public Interest, "New American Eating Guide" (a color poster food guide very similar to the food charts provided in this book), CSPI, 1501 16th Street, Washington, DC 20036.

14. Jane Brody, *Nutrition Book*, p. 222.

15. Dennis Remington, M.D., Garth Fisher, and Edward Parent, *How to Lower Your Fat Thermostat* (Provo, Utah: Vitality House International, 1983), p. 26.

16. Jane Brody, *Nutrition Book*, pp. 245–248.

17. *Consumer Reports* (February), vol. 53, no. 2 (N.Y.: Consumers Union, 1988), pp. 98–99.

18. Ibid.

CHAPTER 9

1. Herbert Greene and Catherine Jones, *Diary of a Food Addict* (N.Y.: Grosset and Dunlap, 1974).

2. A phrase from the 'first of Overeaters Anonymous's twelve steps: *OA Is Not a Diet Club* (pamphlet), Overeaters Anonymous, P.O. Box 92870, Los Angeles, CA 90009.

3. Jon Leonard, Nathaniel Pritikin, and Jack Hoffer, *Live Longer Now* (N.Y.: Grosset and Dunlap, 1974).

Dennis Remington, M.D., Garth Fisher, and Edward Parent, *How to Lower Your Fat Thermostat* (Provo, Utah: Vitality House International, 1983).

4. Betsy Rose, "Coming Into My Years" (BMI).

This refers to a new, *unrecorded* verse. The earlier version of the song is recorded on Betsy's album "Live from the Very Front Row" (Paper Crane Records, Box 79, Cambridge, MA 02238).

RESOURCES

1. Leo Buscaglia, *Living, Loving, and Learning* (N.Y.: Holt, Rinehart and Winston, 1982).

INDEX

Index

Index